ADVANCES IN THE BIOSCIENCES

Volume 58

BRAIN TUMORS: BIOPATHOLOGY AND THERAPY

ADVANCES IN THE BIOSCIENCES

Latest volumes in the series:

BRAIN TUMORS: BIOPATHOLOGY AND THERAPY

Proceedings of the Brain Tumor Workshop —
Verona 1 held in Verona on 13–14 June 1985

Editors:

M. A. GEROSA
M. L. ROSENBLUM
G. TRIDENTE

PERGAMON PRESS

OXFORD · NEW YORK · TORONTO · SYDNEY · FRANKFURT

U.K.   Pergamon Press Ltd., Headington Hill Hall,
                         Oxford OX3 0BW, England

U.S.A.   Pergamon Press Inc., Maxwell House, Fairview Park,
                         Elmsford, New York 10523, U.S.A.

CANADA   Pergamon Press Canada Ltd., Suite 104,
                         150 Consumers Road, Willowdale, Ontario M2J 1P9, Canada

AUSTRALIA   Pergamon Press (Aust.) Pty. Ltd., P.O. Box 544,
                         Potts Point, N.S.W. 2011, Australia

FEDERAL REPUBLIC   Pergamon Press GmbH, Hammerweg 6,
OF GERMANY   D-6242 Kronberg, Federal Republic of Germany

JAPAN   Pergamon Press Ltd., 8th Floor, Matsuoka Central Building,
                         1-7-1 Nishishinjuku, Shinjuku-ku, Tokyo 160, Japan

BRAZIL   Pergamon Editora Ltda., Rua Eça de Queiros, 346,
                         CEP 04011, São Paulo, Brazil

PEOPLE'S REPUBLIC   Pergamon Press, Qianmen Hotel, Beijing,
OF CHINA   People's Republic of China

Contents

Contents

PART TWO : TOPICS IN NEURO-ONCOLOGY

PART THREE : TOPICS IN BRAIN TUMOR THERAPY

PART ONE

TOPICS IN GENERAL ONCOLOGY

Methodologies for *in Vitro* Growth of Human 'Solid' Tumours and Their Applications

B. T. Hill

Laboratory of Cellular Chemotherapy, Imperial Cancer Research Fund, Lincoln's Inn Fields, London WC2A 3PX, UK

Over the last decade there have been significant advances in our knowledge of the growth requirements of human 'solid' tumours, with the result that many laboratory groups have described successful growth of human tumour cells in vitro. Much of the impetus for this work derives from publications by Salmon and his colleagues. In 1977 they reported the development of an in vitro soft agar clonogenic assay suitable for cultivating human tumour cells from fresh biopsy specimens (Hamburger and Salmon, 1977). One year later they provided evidence that this procedure could be used to quantitate the differential sensitivities of these human tumour 'stem' cells to anticancer drugs in vitro, and the results appeared to correlate with patients' clinical responses (Salmon et al, 1978). However, as well as direct agar culture, there are a number of longer term procedures which permit examination of other facets of human tumours: for example, with organ culture the integrity of the three-dimensional cellular interrelationships are retained, multicellular spheroids provide a system of complexity intermediate between 'solid' tumours and the more conventional monolayer or suspension cultures, which in turn offer the major advantage of a continuous supply of cells for experimentation all derived from the same tumour. In this overview each of these methodologies will be considered briefly, attempting to highlight their specific advantages and disadvantages. Their potential applications will then be discussed with particular reference to in vitro drug sensitivity testing, providing examples, where possible, from brain tumour research.

METHODOLOGIES FOR IN VITRO GROWTH OF HUMAN 'SOLID' TUMOURS

As shown in Figure 1, once a human tumour sample is obtained there are a number of different approaches which can be adopted to try and establish in vitro growth.

Organ Culture:
              This technique, applicable to 'solid' tumour specimens involves the maintenance or growth of tissue in vitro to allow differentiation and preservation of architecture and/or function (Schaeffer, 1979). The main advantage of organ culture lies in the fact that structural and functional integrity are maintained. A major limitation, however, is that within these heterogeneous tumour explants there is no qualitative means of distinguishing the response of tumour cells, particularly the 'stem' cells, from the rest of the cellular constituents. Therefore organ culture has been used predominantly for morphological studies or evaluations of hormonal responses in 'hormone-

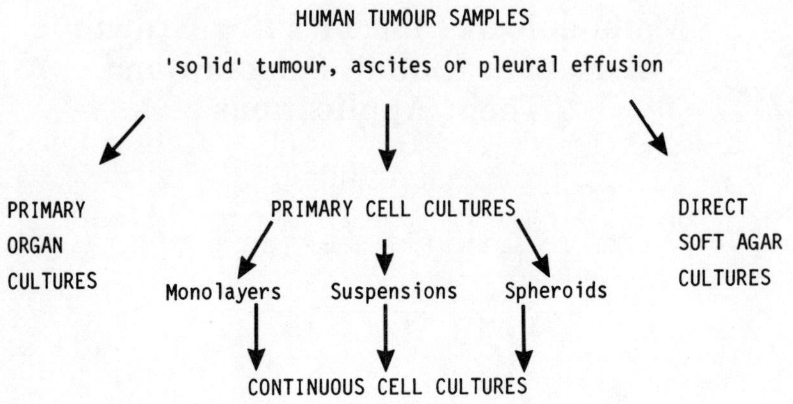

HUMAN TUMOUR SAMPLES

'solid' tumour, ascites or pleural effusion

PRIMARY   PRIMARY CELL CULTURES   DIRECT

ORGAN   SOFT AGAR

CULTURES   Monolayers   Suspensions   Spheroids   CULTURES

CONTINUOUS CELL CULTURES

Figure 1.   Laboratory procedures for in vitro growth of human
            tumour cells.

sensitive' tumours such as breast, prostate and endometrium.   This topic was
reviewed recently by Masters (1983).   There have been several publications
concerning gliomas and neuroblastomas but these have generally been short-term
biological studies (Rubinstein, 1973; Holmstrom, 1975; Sorour et al, 1975
Lyser, 1976): only a few attempts to monitor in vitro drug sensitivities have
been reported (Saez et al, 1977; Darling et al, 1984).

Direct Soft Agar Culture:
                          The most widely used procedure is the bilayer agar
system described by Hamburger and Salmon in 1977, although other groups,
particularly outside North America, favour the alternative replenishable liquid
top soft agar assay devised by Courtenay (1983).   Both of these procedures were
designed specifically for use as in vitro drug sensitivity assays.   Both methods
involve disaggregation of the tumour into a single cell suspension, which is
then exposed to selected concentrations of antitumour agents under defined
conditions, followed by plating into a nutrient agar mixture and subsequent
incubation at 37°C until colonies form which can be counted.   These methodologies, while superficially appearing straightforward have been fraught with
technical problems.   The major centres, predominantly in North America, now
report successful growth in the soft agar colony assay of at least 60% of
specimens, with melanomas and ovarian tumours growing particularly well with a
success rate of 70-80%.   There have been relatively few reports of the use of
these procedures with neurological tumours.   Rosenblum et al, (1981) developed
a variation of the clonogenic assay for human brain tumours and reported
successful growth with 13 malignant gliomas and 8 astrocytomas.   Clark and Von
Hoff (1983), using the Salmon and Hamburger technique, obtained growth suitable
for drug sensitivity testing in only 46% of 114 specimens of brain tumours
plated.   However there have been two more enthusiastic recent preliminary

TABLE I: CURRENT PROBLEMS ASSOCIATED WITH HUMAN TUMOUR
CLONOGENIC ASSAYS

---

1. Not all human tumours grow under these conditions and
there is a need to select carefully the tumour material
for study.

2. Many 'solid' tumours cannot be adequately dissociated
to provide the mandatory 'single cell suspension.

3. Colony forming efficiencies are frequently very low
(0.001-0.1%) so that conditions for optimizing colony
formation need to be established.

4. Questionable growth of 'normal' as well as 'malignant'
cells under these conditions necessitates rigorous
characterization of cells in colonies.

---

reports of success. From 16 malignant glioma specimens, 102 stem cell assays
for drug testing were performed (Georges et al, 1984) and with 59 malignant
brain tumour samples, 48(81%) grew more than 5 colonies and 38(64%) grew over 30
colonies per plate (Mulne et al, 1984). In spite of this though it must be
remembered that the colony forming efficiencies obtained, even at the major
centres, remain exceedingly low, being predominantly of the order of 0.001-0.1%.
Some of the reasons for these problems and failures can perhaps be appreciated
by remembering that these clonogenic assay methodologies require that the
following conditions are rigorously met: (i) the tumour material must be
disaggregated into a 'viable' single cell suspension, so that the clonogenic
cells will then grow from a single cell into a colony, (ii) there must be a
reproducible linear relationship between the number of cells plated into the
agar and the number of colonies formed with each tumour sample. However, in our
experience, and confirmed by Tveit and his colleagues (1983) working with
gliomas, we have consistently obtained improved colony forming efficiencies and
improved colony quality using the Courtenay as opposed to the Hamburger and
Salmon methodology. This has resulted in a higher proportion of samples with
positive colony growth, and the improved quality greatly facilitates manual
colony counting and has aided the plucking of individual colonies for subsequent
analyses of clonal tumour cell populations. Even so the colony forming
efficiencies obtained remain low, generally less than 0.1%, so that growth
conditions for optimising colony formation need to be established.

The main advantages of this type of technology are that fresh biopsy specimens
can be dealt with directly and that the crucially important clonogenic cell
populations, considered to be responsible for maintaining the continued
integrity and growth of the tumour, can be identified and studied. However many
problems remain with these methodologies, as listed in Table I.

These clonogenic assay procedures have been used, not only for in vitro drug
sensitivity testing (see below), but also for studies investigating the biology
of tumours, involving measurements of self renewal capacity, growth modulation
factors, tumour cell heterogeneity and cytogenetics. In these latter respects
the studies of Shapiro and her colleagues working with human gliomas are of
major significance. Initially they demonstrated that some clonal subpopulations rapidly generated new mutant cell types whilst others retained the
parental cell type for at least 3-4 months in culture (Shapiro and Shapiro,
1983). The stable phenotypes were clones that had chromosome numbers in the
near diploid range (40-54 chromosomes), while those that were more prone to

segregational errors had chromosome numbers of 55 or more. Data from their
more recent studies (Shapiro et al, 1984) suggest that it is the near diploid
cells in both parental and clonal populations of a tumour that are the most
resistant to clinically-achievable blood plasma levels of the drug BCNU, whilst
the triploid and tetraploid populations are most sensitive. Therefore they have
concluded that the 'stem' cells of most concern are the near diploid cells that
remain and are the most likely to repopulate the tumour following clinical
intervention.

Primary Cell Cultures:
                            Human tumour biopsy specimens can be disaggregated by a
variety of different techniques, involving either mechanical and/or enzymatic
procedures, and the resulting 'cell suspension' can be plated directly into a
suitable culture vessel. This material can then be used for short-term studies.
One of the main advantages stressed for these primary cultures is that they are
more representative of the tumour from which they were derived than cell lines,
since less time has elapsed since explanation, so there is less opportunity for
selective overgrowth and phenotypic alteration. Subculturing of many carcinomas
often results in loss of the epithelial component and accelerated overgrowth by
stromal cells (Freshney and Dendy, 1983). However, the value of this type of
experimental system is limited by the fact that frequently only a restricted
quantity of material is available, the heterogeneity of cell type plated out may
result in fluctuating growth capacities and there is the questionable influence
of 'normal' cell contaminants. To try and overcome these problems subculture
may be necessary (i) to increase cell numbers to provide sufficient replicates,
and (ii) to provide a greater uniformity of cell type and growth capacity
essential for most types of assay with a biochemical end point to measure
survival. In this way more material can be made available either for short-term
assays, and these have been used in drug sensitivity testing (see below), or for
more long-term studies involving the establishment of continuous human tumour
cell lines.

Continuous Cell Lines:
                            Primary or metastatic tumours, bone marrow aspirations
and pleural effusions have all provided useful material for developing cell
lines. Disaggregated tumour cells can be maintained in suspension culture or
grown as cell monolayers or as multicellular spheroids. Gliomas and neuroblastomas are usually established as monolayer cultures or as multicellular
spheroids (Shapiro et al, 1981; Biedler et al, 1983; Carlsson et al, 1983;
Darling et al, 1983; Nederman, 1983; Schold et al, 1984).

Within the last decade most major tumour types have been established in monolayer culture as continuous cell lines. Success rates of 1-10% are frequently
reported for establishing human tumour cell lines (Smith and Dolbach, 1981), so
there is obviously room for improvement. Problems encountered have included
inadequate tumour sampling, overgrowth by fibroblasts, suboptimal growth
conditions relating to essential concentrations of basal salts or specific
growth factors, and the use of only plastic or glass substrates. A detailed
characterisation of the lines once they are established is absolutely essential,
particularly ensuring their human origin by chromosome and isozyme analyses and
confirming the absence of cell contaminants such as HeLa cells. We also carry
out examination by light and electromicroscopy and, where appropriate, attempt
immunological identification using monoclonal antibodies. The tumourogenicity
of the lines is established by evaluating growth in soft agar and/or as xeno-
grafts in nude mice. The chief advantage of cell monolayers is that they
provide a readily available source of cells, all derived from the same tumour,
which permit both reproducible and reliable experimental data to be obtained.
Continuous cell lines have been used in studies of the biology of human tumours,
identifying growth modulation factors, for the development of monoclonal antibodies and for drug sensitivity evaluations (discussed below). However, it must
be remembered that such cell lines represent discrete subpopulations within a

heterogeneous tumour specimen, characterised by their capacity for vigorous and maintained growth under in vitro conditions. It remains to be established whether these are truly representative of the 'stem cell populations' of tumours growing in vivo.

This same reservation, of course, applies to the use of multicellular spheroids. Spheroids consist of aggregated cells in a spherical configuration. Peripheral cells proliferate intensively and contribute to spheroid growth. Deeper lying cells probably suffer from a poor supply of nutrients and inadequate clearance of catabolic products and so proliferation decreases as a function of depth. The chief advantage of this particular technique is that it allows a simulation of the drug penetration barrier which may exist in poorly vascularized regions of 'solid' tumours and of the proliferation gradients and different micro-environments within these tumours. Therefore experimental studies with human tumour spheroids have centred on: (i) drug penetration studies, (ii) proliferation-dependent cytotoxic effects of drugs and (iii) models for investigating drug resistance (for example, see reviews by Sutherland et al, 1981 and Nederman, 1983).

IN VITRO DRUG SENSITIVITY TESTING USING HUMAN TUMOUR MATERIAL

Studies aimed at devising an in vitro drug sensitivity test applicable to individual patients' tumour samples, for predicting suitable chemotherapy, have employed both primary tumour biopsy material and continuous cell lines. This work has been reviewed extensively (for example, see Hamburger, 1981; Livingston, 1981; Von Hoff et al, 1981; Weisenthal et al, 1981; Salmon, 1982). In this brief overview I would like to highlight only a few specific aspects.

When attempting to devise a suitable in vitro drug sensitivity test the end point used to assess the cytotoxic effects of drugs has first to be selected. For 'short-term' assays, providing results in a few days, three main types of procedure have been used: vital dye exclusion, counting tumour cell numbers or incorporation of radioactive nucleic acid or protein precursors. The use of clonogenic or colony-forming assays involves more 'long-term' evaluation, since depending on the tumour type colonies take between ten days and six weeks to form and provide a definitive end-point. The advantages and disadvantages of these different test procedures have been reviewed (Hill, 1983a). A more recent development involves a rapid test based on tritiated thymidine incorporation in soft-agar culture (Tanigawa et al, 1982). Results of this assay correlated with chemosensitivities determined by the soft-agar clonogenic assay. A miniaturized version of this procedure has recently been reported to give a high evaluability rate for most common human 'solid' tumours, it required fewer tumour cells for each assay and the result was obtained within five days (Kern et al, 1985).

A simple 'short-term' test has obvious advantages over the time-consuming and labour intensive clonogenic assays. However, as shown in a number of studies, the clonogenic assay remains the most reliable predictor of tumour cell survival (Roper and Drewinko, 1976; Rupniak et al, 1983). We measured the effects of four antitumour drugs (methotrexate, vincristine, cis-platinum and adriamycin) on tumour cell survival comparing results from two 'short-term' procedures based upon dye exclusion and labelling index determinations with data from colony-forming assays. Data for cis-platinum and adriamycin are illustrated in Figure 2. The dye exclusion procedure showed the poorest correlation with the clonogenic assay, whereas labelling index measurements exhibited qualitative, if not quantitative, correspondence with results from the clonogenic assays. These 'short-term' procedures therefore cannot be considered accurate substitutes for measurements of reproductive cell survival. We consider that the clonogenic assay remains the method of choice for assessing cytotoxic effects of antitumour drugs.

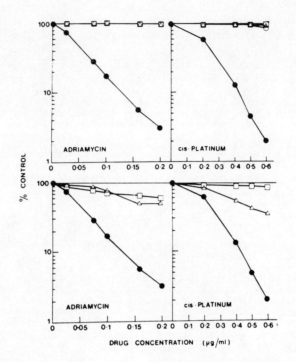

Figure 2. TOP PANELS - Comparison of cell survival as assessed
by colony-forming assay (●) and a dye exclusion
assay performed at 24 hr (□), 48 hr (△) or 72 hr (○)
after drug addition.
BOTTOM PANELS - Comparison of cell survival as
assessed by colony-forming assay (●) and a
labelling index assay performed over the periods
24-48 hr (□) and 48-72 hr (△) after drug addition.

(Reproduced in part from Rupniak et al, 1983 with
permission from the first author and the Director
of 'Tumori'.)

TABLE II: CRITERIA FOR SUCCESSFUL APPLICATION OF HUMAN
            TUMOUR CLONOGENIC ASSAYS

Clonogenic assay methodologies require that the following conditions
are rigorously met:

1.   the tumour material must be disaggregated into a 'viable'
        single cell suspension, so that the clonogenic cells will
        then produce a colony from a single cell,

2.   there must be a reproducible linear relationship between
        the number of cells plated into the agar and the number
        of colonies formed, for each tumour specimen,

3.   there must be adequate colony formation so that following
        exposure of the tumour cells to a drug a quantitative
        assessment of its cytotoxic effects on tumour cell survival
        is possible.

Successful application of the clonogenic assay methodologies to provide a
reliable in vitro drug evaluation requires, however, that a number of necessary
conditions are rigourously met. These are listed in Table II. Unfortunately
failure to meet one or all of these criteria is frequently reported so that
between 30-50% of samples received for testing prove to be unassessable. To
increase the success rate superior methods for 'solid' tumour disaggregation,
perhaps involving different enzyme 'cocktails' as discussed by Hill (1983b),
must be defined and improved colony-forming efficiencies must be obtained. At
present, if we assume a colony-forming efficiency of 0.01%, require at least 30
colonies in control sample dishes, set up samples in triplicate and test three
drug concentrations for a single in vitro exposure duration, a minimum of 3.6
million tumour cells would be needed for each drug test. Clearly enhancing the
colony forming efficiency by 10- or even 100-fold would allow us not only to
derive more reliable dose response curves, but also to evaluate a larger number
of drugs over a range of concentrations and drug exposure durations for single
agents and for combinations. In addition, this would further reduce the number
of inevaluable tumour specimens. Achievement of this improvement in colony
forming ability will almost certainly involve manipulation of culture conditions
and their more precise tuning for individual tumour types. Furthermore,
specific growth requirements may more easily be met by using chemically-defined
media, which are already available for a number of cell lines derived from, for
example, lymphomas, bladder, breast, neuroblastoma, lung and prostate tumours
(as reviewed earlier, Hill, 1983c), but not yet for brain tumours. Indeed,
improvements in techniques for culturing brain tumours in vitro will benefit
not only groups employing clonogenic assay tests, but also those using multicellular spheroids or primary monolayer cultures for cytotoxicity evaluations.

LABORATORY AND CLINICAL CORRELATIONS OF DRUG SENSITIVITIES

Irrespective of the in vitro test procedure adopted, or the criteria used to
define sensitivity, the main conclusion that can be drawn from studies with all
types of human tumour specimens is that these methodologies appear useful for
predicting drug resistance accurately. This observation also appears to hold
for the limited number of such studies reported using neurological tumours (see
Table III). This conclusion has led to one of the criticisms commonly levelled
at these in vitro drug tests, namely that they fail to provide a sensitivity
test and only predict resistance. Since a large majority of these studies have
been carried out on biopsies from previously-treated patients who have relapsed,

TABLE III: LABORATORY AND CLINICAL CORRELATIVE STUDIES
INVOLVING IN VITRO DRUG SENSITIVITY TESTING
OF NEUROLOGICAL TUMOURS

Assay Method	No. & Type of Tumours	% Correlations of Sensitivity	Resistance	Reference
Cell counting	13 astrocytomas (grades III & IV)	63% (5/8)	100% (5/5)	Kornblith et al. 1981
Clonogenic assay	15 glioblastomas	43% (3/7)	100% (8/8)	Rosenblum et al. 1981
35 S-methionine uptake	40 gliomas (grades III & IV)	In vitro sensitivity in 55% correlated with significantly longer relapse-free intervals		Thomas et al. 1985

this finding rather than demeaning the value of the assays tends instead to be a point in their favour, since this group of patients are known clinically to have disease largely refractory to present chemotherapy. Furthermore, by accurately defining drugs to which the patient is unlikely to respond, unnecessary chemotherapy may be avoided. However, the fact remains that it is only a small minority of patients for whom an active drug can be identified using these in vitro tests; taking all the tumour types evaluated in many thousands of such tests the sensitivity figure approximates to 10%. Although the data in Table III suggests that sensitivity may be predicted accurately in approximately 50% of patients with neurological tumours, this figure may well prove optimistic since the number of tumours tested in these studies are small (<100) and almost certainly there was patient selection. However, there does appear to be an interesting correlation between in vitro sensitivity of gliomas and clinical response using the intermediate duration cytotoxicity assay (Darling and Thomas, 1983; Thomas et al, 1985). These data therefore, should provide encouragement for prospective clinical trials to be carried out and since there is a need for a large input of patients into each trial it may well be necessary to set up multicentre studies.

RECENT DEVELOPMENTS AND FUTURE PROSPECTS

Whilst accepting the requirements for new and improved methodologies, for more data supporting the validity of present assay methodologies and, especially, for prospective clinical trials preferable assessing results in terms of survival rather than response to chemotherapy, we can still expand our horizons using technology presently available. There are a number of potential clinical applications of these in vitro tests. Those relating particularly to clonogenic assays are listed in Table IV.

My laboratory has been interested in one of these applications, namely investigating the scheduling of antitumour drugs. In initial studies, using ovarian tumour biopsy material and the Courtenay clonogenic assay, we evaluated sensitivities to adriamycin and cisplatin. We consistently observed increased cell kill with increasing drug concentrations but also, were able to show that enhanced cell kill resulted from prolonging the in vitro exposure duration beyond one hour (Rupniak et al, 1983). In subsequent studies (Hill et al, 1984),

TABLE IV: POTENTIAL CLINICAL APPLICATIONS OF THESE
             CLONOGENIC ASSAY PROCEDURES

---

1.   In vitro Phase II testing of 'new' agents.

2.   Initial screening of antitumour drug analogues.

3.   Optimising scheduling of antitumour drugs.

4.   Establishing patterns of cross resistance and
      collateral sensitivity for 'old' and 'new' drugs,
      so as to identify drugs potentially useful for
      treating relapsing patients.

5.   Monitoring the development of drug resistance in
      patients' tumours, when serial biopsies are
      available.

6.   Determining the relationship between clonogenicity
      and prognosis.

7.   Tumour detection in bone marrow samples.

---

we have confirmed and extended there findings and highlighted the facts that
(i) duration of exposure is an important determinant of drug-induced cytotoxicity under these assay conditions, and (ii) that employing only a one hour
drug exposure is inadequate for evaluating the cytotoxic effects of certain
drugs, including vincristine, hydroxyurea and VP-16-213. These data therefore
indicate that the use of a single set of "standard" drug exposure conditions for
in vitro drug sensitivity testing is likely to be inappropriate, particularly
when testing new agents without knowledge of their pharmacokinetic properties.
Furthermore, these results suggest that benefit may accrue clinically by
changing the way in which "standard" antitumour drugs are administered and
extending the duration of drug treatment (Hill et al, 1985).

The other applications listed in Table IV are also being investigated in a
number of laboratories, although at the present time few are being applied to
neurological tumour samples. Friedman et al, (1984) have recently reported the
in vitro chemosensitivity of a human medulloblastoma cell line TE-671 using a
clonogenic assay and have shown how these data can be correlated with results of
xenograft growth delay produced by the same drugs in the athymic mouse model.
Whilst suggesting that this in vitro - in vivo model may allow screening of
agents effective against medulloblastoma, they also stress that tumour heterogeneity would argue against the use of only one continuous cell line.   Indeed,
Yung et al, (1982) were one of the first groups to identify heterogeneity of
chemosensitivities among subpopulations of human malignant glioma cells in
culture, when testing BCNU and cis-platinum. These authors emphasized the need
to consider such variability when designing chemotherapy programmes and
cautioned against interpretation of tests on individual patients' tumour samples
in the light of this inherent heterogeneity.

It is therefore probable that in the next decade there will be a shift in
emphasis, away from the idea of predicting and tailoring chemotherapy programmes
for individual patients using these in vitro test procedures, towards studies
which will provide more general information which may lead not only to the
identification of new drugs for specific tumour types but also to the optimal
scheduling of the antitumour drugs already in clinical use. In this way it is

hoped therefore that fruitful collaborative research programmes will continue
and new ones will be initiated so that their full clinical potential can be
exploited.

ACKNOWLEDGEMENTS

I am extremely grateful to John L. Darling and John R.W. Masters for helpful
advice and discussions during the preparation of this manuscript. The valuable
secretarial assistance of Alison Barrow was much appreciated.

REFERENCES

Biedler, J.L., M.B. Meyers and B.A. Spengler (1983). Adv. Cell. Neurobiol., 4,
267-307.
Carlsson J., K. Nilsson, B. Westermark, J. Ponten, C. Sundstrom, E. Larsson,
J. Bergh, S. Pahlman, C. Busch and V.P. Collins (1983). Int. J. Cancer, 31,
523-533.
Clark, G.M. and D.D. Von Hoff (1983). Human Tumour Drug Sensitivity Testing In
Vitro, Eds. P.P. Dendy and B.T. Hill, pp. 225-233, Academic Press, London.
Courtenay, D. (1983). Human Tumour Drug Sensitivity Testing In Vitro, Eds.
P.P. Dendy and B.T. Hill, pp. 103-111, Academic Press, London.
Darling, J.L. and D.G.T. Thomas (1983). Human Tumour Drug Sensitivity Testing
In Vitro, Eds. P.P. Dendy and B.T. Hill, pp. 269-280, Academic Press, London.
Darling, J.L., N. Oktar and D.G.T. Thomas (1983). Cell. Biol. Int. Rep., 7,
23-30.
Darling, J.L., J.R.W. Masters and N.J. Bradley (1984). J. Neuro. Oncol., 2, 291.
Freshney, R.I. and P.P. Dendy (1983). Human Tumour Drug Sensitivity Testing In
Vitro, Eds. P.P. Dendy and B.T. Hill, pp. 69-89, Academic Press, London.
Friedman, H.S., S.C. Schold, L.H. Muhlbaier, T.D. Bjornsson and D.D. Bigner
(1984). Cancer Res., 44, 5145-5149.
Georges, P.M., C. Sanders, W. Rombaut, M. Rosensweig and J. Brotchi (1984).
J. Neuro. Oncol., 2, 287.
Hamburger, A.W. (1981). J. Natl. Cancer Inst., 66, 981-988.
Hamburger, A.W. and S.E. Salmon (1977). Science, 197, 461-463.
Hill, B.T. (1983a). Human Tumour Drug Sensitivity Testing In Vitro, Eds.
P.P. Dendy and B.T. Hill, pp. 235-249, Academic Press, London.
Hill, B.T. (1983b). Human Tumour Drug Sensitivity Testing In Vitro, Eds.
P.P. Dendy and B.T. Hill, pp. 91-102, Academic Press, London.
Hill, B.T. (1983c). Human Tumour Drug Sensitivity Testing In Vitro, Eds.
P.P. Dendy and B.T. Hill, pp. 129-146, Academic Press, London
Hill, B.T., R.D.H. Whelan, L.K. Hosking, B.G. Ward and E.M. Gibby (1984).
Human Tumor Cloning, Eds. S.E. Salmon and J.M. Trent, pp. 487-496, Grune and
Stratton, Inc., Orlando.
Hill, B.T., R.D.H. Whelan and E.M. Gibby (1985). Proc. Am. Assoc. Cancer Res.,
26, 362.
Holmstrom, T. (1975). Human Tumor Cells In Vitro, Ed. J. Fogh, pp. 161-174,
Plenum Press, New York.
Kern, D.H., C.R. Drogemuller, M.C. Kennedy, S.U. Hildebrand-Zanki and
N. Tanigawa (1985). Cancer Res., 45, in press.
Kornblith, P.L., B.H. Smith and L.A. Leonard (1981). Cancer, 47, 255-265.
Livingston, R.B. (1981). Breast Cancer. IV. Advances in Research and Treatment,
Ed. W.L. McGuire, pp. 1-32, Plenum Press, New York.
Lyser, K.M. (1976). In Vitro, 12, 48-56.
Masters, J.R.W. (1983). Human Tumour Drug Sensitivity Testing In Vitro,
Eds. P.P. Dendy and B.T. Hill, pp. 163-177, Academic Press, London.
Mulne, A.F., M.L. Salgaller, A.J. Yates and P.D. Walson (1984). Proc. Am. Assoc.
Cancer Res., 25, 29.
Nederman, T. (1983). Human Tumour Drug Sensitivity Testing In Vitro,
Eds. P.P. Dendy and B.T. Hill, pp. 147-161, Academic Press, London.
Roper, P. and B. Drewinko (1976). Cancer Res., 36, 2182-2188.

Roper, P. and B. Drewinko (1976). Cancer Res., 36, 2182-2188.
Rosenblum, M.L., D.V. Dougherty, C. Reese and C.B. Wilson (1981). Cancer
    Chemother. Pharmacol., 6, 227-235.
Rubinstein, L.J., M.M. Herman and V.L. Foley (1973). Am. J. Path., 71, 61-80.
Rupniak, H.T., L.Y. Dennis and B.T. Hill (1983a). Tumori, 69, 37-42.
Rupniak, H.T., R.D.H. Whelan and B.T. Hill (1983b). Int. J. Cancer, 32, 7-12.
Saez, R.J., R.J. Campbell and E.R. Laws (1977). J. Neurosurg., 46, 320-327.
Salmon, S.E. (1983). Human Tumour Drug Sensitivity Testing In Vitro,
    Eds. P.P. Dendy and B.T. Hill, pp. 291-303, Academic Press, London.
Salmon, S.E., A.W. Hamburger, B. Soehnlen, B.G.M. Durie, D.S. Alberts and
    T.E. Moon (1978). New Engl. J. Med., 298, 1321-1327.
Schaeffer, W.I. (1979). In Vitro, 15, 649-653.
Shapiro, J.R., W-K.A. Yung and W.R. Shapiro (1981). Cancer Res., 41, 2349-2359.
Shapiro, J.R. and W.R. Shapiro (1983). Rational Basis For Chemotherapy,
    Ed. B.A. Chabner, pp. 45-59, Alan R. Liss, Inc., New York.
Shapiro, J.R., P-Y. Pu and W.R. Shapiro (1984). Human Tumor Cloning, Eds.
    S.E. Salmon and J.M. Trent, pp. 133-142, Grune and Stratton, Inc., Orlando.
Schold, S.C., H.S. Friedman, T.D. Bjornsson and D.D. Bigner (1984). Cancer
    Res., 44, 2352-2357.
Smith, H.S. and C.M. Dollbaum (1981). Tissue Growth Factors, Ed. R. Baserga,
    pp. 451-490. Springer Verlag, Berlin.
Sorour, O., M. Raafat, N. El-Bolkainy and M. Rifaat (1975). J. Neurosurg., 43,
    742-749.
Sutherland, R.M., J. Carlsson, R. Durand and J. Yuhas (1981). Cancer Res., 41,
    2980-2984.
Tanigawa, N., D.H. Kern, Y. Hikasa and D.L. Morton (1982). Cancer Res., 44,
    2159-2164.
Thomas, D.G.T., J.L. Darling, E.A. Paul, T.J. Mott, J.N. Godlee, J.S. Tobias,
    L.G. Capra, C.D. Collins, C. Mooney, T. Bozek, G.P. Finn, S.O. Arigbabu,
    D.E. Bullard, N. Shannon and R.I. Freshney (1985). Br. J. Cancer, 51,
    525-532.
Tveit, K.M., L. Endresen, S. Gundersen, S. Vaage, M. Davy, H.E. Rugstad and
    A. Pihl (1983). Proc. 13th Int. Congress of Chemotherapy, Eds. K.H. Spitzy
    and K. Karrer, Part 224, 9-14.
Von Hoff, D.D., J. Casper, E. Bradley, J. Sandbach, D. Jones and R. Makuch
    (1981). Am. J. Med., 70, 1027-1032.
Weisenthal, L.N., J.A. Marsden, P.L. Dill and C.K. Macaluso (1983). Cancer
    Res., 43, 749-757.
Yung, W-K.A., J.R. Shapiro and W.R. Shapiro (1982). Cancer Res., 42, 992-998.

Cell Kinetic Studies in Solid Tumors

E. Di Marco*, A. Nicolin*, A. Alama*
and P. F. Conte**

*Department of Pharmacology, Istituto Nazionale per la Ricerca
sul Cancro, Genova, Italy
**Division of Medical Oncology, Istituto Nazionale per la Ricerca
sul Cancro, Genova, Italy

Research supported by CNR, Special Project "Oncology"
Contract No. 84.00529.44, Rome, Italy

ABSTRACT

Cell kinetic has assumed a remarkable prognostic relevance in human tumors, included
those affecting the CNS. In this laboratory tumor cell kinetic is under study in a
number of solid tumors by two experimental assays: The Thymidine Labeling Index
(TLI) and the Primer Dependent DNA Polymerase (PDP) that indicate S phase cells or
growth fraction (GF), respectively.
Growth fraction evaluation plays a major role in understanding the kinetic features of
individual tumors. Previous experimental approaches were laborious and ethycally
questionable. Moreover, failure to cure in cancer chemotherapy (CT) is due to
permanent or temporary chemoresistance. It is well known that resting tumor cells are
more resistant to CT than corresponding proliferating cells thus surviving drug
treatment. The recruitment of resting cells into the proliferative pool has been
performed in locally advanced breast cancer treated with 1 mg diethylstilbestrol (DES)
to increase cells sensitivity to CT. By TLI assay and PDP assay it was demostrated the
actual recruitment of tumor cells independently of ER content of tumor cells, leading
to effective response to conventional CT.
This cytokinetic approach to cancer chemotherapy, if definitely confirmed, might be
extended to tumors other than mammary provided specific recruiting agents are used.

INTRODUCTION

Availability since 1957 of tritium labeled precursor of DNA synthesis has greately
improved the knowledge of kinetic parameters of experimental and human tumors.
From the large amount of experimental data so far available, three striking
characteristics of tumor growth are apparent:

1) The percentage of proliferating tumor cells (growth fraction) is usually lower than the normal counterpart (Steel, 1977); this kinetic finding is apparently conflicting with the restless growth of tumors in comparison with the ordered and limited growth of normal tissues. In fact tumors grow continuously, despite a usually lower growth fraction, because cancer cells have lost the capacity to differentiate, therefore most non-proliferating cancer cells can re-enter the cell cycle (Gabutti, et al., 1969). Moreover normal cells start proliferation because triggered by specific growth factors (i.c. erythropoietin for red cells precursors) while tumor cell proliferation is relatively independent by host regulatory mechanisms.

2) There is no "typical" characteristic of tumor growth, in fact the only "common" kinetic parameter is the great heterogeneity in the percentage of S phase cells in tumors of the same histologic type.

3) Most antiblastic drugs exert their maximal cytocidal efficacy on proliferating cells. (Drewinko, et al., 1981).

The relevance of these data for clinicians dealing with cancer is dual:

a) Difference in kinetic parameters can account for the commonly observed different prognosis in patients with tumors of the same histotype and stage. In fact the percentage of thymidine labeled cells (TLI) has proved to be a reliable prognostic index in many human tumors (Meyer, et al., 1983; Gentili, et al., 1981; Costa, et al., 1981).

b) Dependence of cell killing upon cell proliferation can be exploited in order to increase the therapeutic index of antiblastic drugs (Hill, 1978.; Conte, et al., 1984; Conte, et al., 1985); if chemotherapy is administered when most cancer cells are proliferating while normal cells are resting the therapeutic effect is maximized and damage on normal tissues reduced.

Unfortunately so far these promising principles of tumor cell kinetics have received little application in the management of human cancer, because the majority of experimental data have been obtained in animal tumors. Technical and ethical considerations in fact have severely limited investigations on human beings. In the present paper we provide evidence that new reliable techniques can overcome this problem thus allowing a more widespread utilization of cell kinetic data in the strategy of cancer therapy.

MATERIALS AND METHODS

Tumor proliferative activity was evaluated by TLI and PDP-LI (see below) in 89 breast cancers, 49 epithelial ovarian carcinomas, 25 colo-rectal carcinomas and 8 squamous cell carcinomas of the head and neck.

In 24 patients with locally advanced breast carcinoma tumor proliferative activity was repetidly evaluated during treatment with diethylstilbestrol (DES 1 mg/die for 3 days) and FAC chemotherapy (5 FU 600 mg/m^2 + Adriamycin 50 mg/m^2 + Cytoxan 600 mg/m^2) on day 4: tumor biopsies were performed before treatment (T_0), after DES (T_1), 24 hrs. after the first FAC (T_2) and at the time of surgery, after 3 DES-FAC (T_3).

Thimidine Labeling Index (TLI).
Tumor cells were obtained by mechanical disaggregation of fresh tumor biopsies; cells were suspended in RPMI 1640 + 10% fetal calf serum (2-3 . 10^6/ml), incubated for 30 min. at 37°C with 10 µCi/ml of ^{3}H d Thd (s.a. 5 Ci/mM Amersham), washed twice in cold saline, cytocentrifuged onto acid-cleaned slides and fixed in methanol-acetic (3:1) for 15 min. Slides were then dipped in Kodak NTB-2 nuclear track emulsion (Eastern Kodak Rochester, NY), exposed for 24 hrs. and submitted to gold activated autoradiography (Braunschweiger, et al., 1973). The labeled cells represent the percentage of S-phase cells.

Primer dependent ⍺ DNA Polymerase Assay (PDP-LI).
The PDP assay detects the simultaneous presence of nuclear ⍺ DNA polymerase and nuclear DNA primer template activity in viable cell nuclei. This ⍺ DNA polymerase is

present in all activity cycling cells, therefore the PDP-LI represents an in vitro measure of tumor growth fraction (Schiffer, et al., 1976). Briefly, fresh tumor cells were suspended in NaCl 0.9% and cytocentrifuged onto slides; thereafter the slides were dipped in 0.25% agar solution at 41-42 °C in order to disrupt the cytoplasm while leaving the intact nuclei on the slides; the nuclei were then incubated for 45 min at 37°C in 5% CO_2 with 0.081 mM each of Deoxyadenosine -5'-Triphosphate; Deoxycytidine-5'-Triphosphate; Deoxyguanosine -5'-Triphosphate (Sigma Chemical Co, St.Louis, Mo) and 10 μCi/ml of ^3H Deoxythymidine -5'-Triphosphate (s.a. 60-80 Ci/mM, New England Nuclear, Boston, Mass.)

Radiolabeling was stopped in cold saline solution, the slides were fixed in Acidic Formaldehyde (100 ml Formalin, 25 ml 1 N HCl, 875 ml water) for 30 min, washed in tap water, dehydratated in Ethanol, Xylene and Acetone.

Finally the slides were dipped in NTB-2 nuclear track emulsion, exposed for 7 days at 4°C and submitted to gold activated autoradiography. The percentage of labeled nuclei (PDP-LI) is an in vitro measure of tumor growth fraction. Further details on the TLI and PDP-LI techniques have been published previously (Conte, et al., 1985).

RESULTS

Mean TLIs and PDP-LIs of human solid tumor are reported in Table 1. Untreated colorectal carcinomas displayed the highest proliferative activity (TLI = 11.6%; PDP-LI = 17.7%) followed by untreated ovarian cancer (TLI = 3.9%; PDP-LI 13.99); proliferative activity of breast and head and neck carcinomas was very similar and far lower than that recorded for colon and ovarian cancer. In all the tumors in study PDP-LI values exceeded TLI values: mean PDP-LI/TLI ratios are 2.3, 2.3, 3.3 and 1.5 in breast, head and neck, ovarian and colon cancer respectively.

Relapsing breast and ovarian carcinomas showed a higher proliferative activity than primary, untreated tumors: this difference is particularly striking for ovarian carcinoma (Table 2). In the 24 patients with locally advanced breast cancer TLI and PDP-LI during treatment were the following:

		T_0	T_1	T_2	T_3
TLI	=	1.8	3.3	1.7	0.8
PDP-LI	=	5.9	8.3	3.2	2.9

Interestingly DES was able to induce an increase in both TLI and PDP-LI (estrogenic recruitment) irrespectively of estrogen receptor status of the tumors.

TABLE 1: In vitro proliferative activity of human solid tumors.

	TLI %	PDP-LI %
Breast Cancer	3.0 (0.2-26.1)	6.8 (0.8-22.8)
Ovarian Cancer	6.0 (0.2-35.0)	19.6 (3.0-65.5)
H & N Cancer	3.0 (0.5- 4.1)	6.8 (1.3-13.2)
Colon Cancer	11.6 (1.0-50.1)	17.7 (3.0-69.6)

TABLE 2: Proliferantive activity of human solid tumors at diagnosis and at relapse.

	TLI (%)	PDP-LI (%)
Primary Ovarian Cancer	3.9	13.99
Relapsing Ovarian Cancer	8.1	29.3
Primary Breast Cancer	3.08	6.4
Relapsing Breast Cancer	2.74	7.9

DISCUSSION

The rate of tumor growth is strictly determined to the clinical outcome of cancer patients: high proliferative activity is associated with severe prognosis in breast cancer, multiple myeloma, non Hodgkin lymphomas and acute leukemias (Meyer, et al., 1983; Gentili, et al., 1981; Costa, et al., 1981; Durie, et al., 1980).
Knowledge of kinetic parameters of human tumors let allow the choice of a more rational strategy of cancer therapy.Furthermore most antiblastic compounds display their optimal citotoxicity on proliferating cells: the same amount of drug can kill different proportions of normal and neoplastic cells according to their proliferative status (Drewinko, et al., 1981).
Unfortunately the principles of cell kinetics have received so far scant application in cancer chemotherapy, mainly because ethical and technical considerations have severely limited a sistematic study in human tumors.
In the present paper we provide evidence that two in vitro techniques can be routinely utilized to evaluate tumor proliferative activity of fresh tumor biopsies.
In particular the PDP assay, so far utilized mainly in experimental tumors, seems promising: this technique, in fact, allows the detection of proliferating cells even if not engaged in the S-phase of the cell-cycle; the PDP-LI is therefore an in vitro measure of tumor growth fraction (Schiffer, et al., 1976).
Evalutation of the growth fraction offers three advantages in comparison to "classic" TLI (which represents the percentage of cells in DNA synthesis):
1) PDP-LI scores are higher than corresponding TLI; therefore differences between showly and rapidly growing tumors are more evident.
2) The PDP depends not only on the number of cells in the S-phase, but also on the lenght of this phase:
the same TLI value could mean a low proportion of cells slowly proceeding along the S-phase or conversely a higher proportion of rapidly cycling cells. On the contrary the PDP-assay can detect all proliferating cells even outside the S-phase, therefore it is less dependent from the cell cycle transit times.
3) The PDP-LI can usefully be exploited to design of cytokinetic chemotherapy because most antiblastic agents are effective preferentially on proliferating cells while only a few drugs are true S-phase specific.
The possibility to exploit cell kinetic parameters for the design of new therapeutic regimens is clearly demonstrated by our data in locally advanced breast cancer: DES was able to recall into the proliferative pool resting cancer cell thus increasing the killing efficiency of subsequently administered chemotherapy.
In conclusion, availability of in vitro techniques such as TLI and PDP-LI will allow a better knowledge of proliferative activity of human solid tumors and, hopefully, will result in a more rational approach to the treatment of human cancer.

REFERENCES

Braunschweiger, P.G., L., Poulakos and M.L., Schiffer (1973).
Cancer Res., 36, 1748-1753.
Conte, P.F., A., Alama, R.E., Favoni, F., Trave, R., Rosso and
A.,Nicolin (1984). Eur. J. Cancer Clin. Oncol., 20, 1039-1043.
Conte, P.F., A., Alama, A., Nicolin, E., Corsaro, G., Canavese, R.,
Rosso, G.,Fraschini and B., Drewinko (1985). Cancer Res., (in press).
Costa, A., G., Bonadonna, E., Villa, P., Valagussa and R., Silvestrini
(1981). J.Natl. Cancer Inst., 66, 1-5.
Drewinko, B., M., Patchen, L. Y., Yang and B., Barlogie (1981).
Cancer Res., 41, 2328-2333.
Durie, B.G.M., S. E., Salmon and T.E. Moon (1980). Blood, 55, 364.
Gabutti, W., A., Pileri, R.P.Tarocco et al. (1969). Nature, 224, 375-
376.
Gentili, C., O.,Sanfilippo and R., Silvestrini (1981). Cancer, 48, 974-
978.
Hill, B.T. (1979). Biochem. Biophys. Acta, 516, 389-417.
Meyer, J.S., E., Friedman, M., Mc Crate and W.C., Bauer (1983).
Cancer, 51, 1979-1981.
Schiffer, M.L., A.M., Markoe and J.S.R., Nelson (1976). Cancer Res,
36, 2415-2418.
Steel, G.G. (1977). Clorendon Press., Oxford.

Translocations and Genetic Rearrangements in Leukemias and Lymphomas

R. Sitia

Laboratory of Molecular Biology, Istituto Nazionale per la Ricerca
sul Cancro, Genoa, Italy

The genetic rearrangements leading to immunoglobulin production
by B lymphocytes and their relationship with the genesis of B cell
malignacies will be briefly reviewed. A murine B lymphoma model
system, which has been studied extensively in our laboratory, will
also be described in the context of certain molecular events of
B cell differentiation and transformation.

A) Structure, Rearrangements and Expression of Immunoglobulin
   Genes .

1) Structure and function of immunoglobulin.

An immunoglobulin molecule is composed of two identical heavy
(H) chains and two identical light (L) chains. Light chains
may be of two types, K and λ , while in the human heavy chains
exist in 9 classes or subclasses (isotypes): $\mu, \delta, \gamma_1, \gamma_2, \gamma_3, \gamma_4, \varepsilon, \alpha_1, \alpha_2$
Three separate genetic loci encode H, K and λ chains. IgH,
IgK and Igλ are located on different chromosomes (14,2,22 in
the human, 12,6,16 in the mouse, respectively). Ig molecules
may be subdivided on the basis of sequence analyses into a
variable (V) and a constant (C) regions. The former, composed
by the NH_2 terminal domains of heavy (V_H) and light (V_L)
chains, mediates the binding with the antigen, while the C
region is responsible of the functional properties of the antibody molecule (complement fixation, binding to cellular Fc
receptors etc.). (1)
The problem of how to reconcile the existence of many (up to
10^8) variable regions with very few constant regions (classical experiments had shown that each C_H gene is present in a
single copy per haploid genome) has puzzled immunologists for
over thirty years. The solution of this problem, made possible
by the fundamental contributions of Susumu Tonegawa, Leroy

Hood, Philip Leder, Cesar Milstein and their associates, has represented a real revolution in modern biology.

2) **Different genes encode V and C regions of immunoglobulin molecules.**

In 1976 Susumu Tonegawa and coworkers demonstrated that distinct genetic elements encode V and C . V_L and C_L are far
from each other in cells which do not produce immunoglobulins,
but undergo a genetic rearrangement which brings them in close
proximity in cells of the B lymphocytic lineage (2). Tonegawa
proposed that the V-C rearrangement not only made possible the
synthesis of Ig molecules, but signaled by itself the activation of Ig transcription and expression. These findings buried
the dogma "one gene - one polypeptide" and implyed that the
genome of the B cell differs from that of the germ line.

FIG. 1

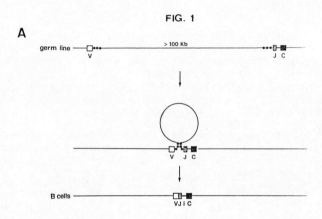

FIGURE 1.The rearrangements of variable and constant region genes for light(A)
          and heavy(B) chains.The dots indicate particular consensus sequences
          that probably mediate the recombination phenomena.In panel B is indi-
          cated the order of C_H genes on mouse chromosome 12. In the human the
          order is: μ -δ -γ_3 -γ_2 -$\psi\varepsilon$-α_1- γ_ε -γ_4 - ε-α_2. The genes for μ and δ are
          much closer to each other than any other C_H gene.There is no S region
          5' to $C\delta$. This explains why most B lymphocytes coexpress μ and δ ,via
          an alternate splicing mechanism.

3) Variable regions are encoded by multiple gene segments.

Further work revealed that the genes encoding the variable regions of L chains are composed by two distinct genetic elements, V_L (variable) and J_L, (joining). The number of V_L genes in the germ line is still unclear, ranging from 30 to 300 in the extimates of several groups, while there exist 5 J_L genes. A third genetic element, termed D (diversity) contributes to form the variable region of heavy chains. It is thought that the germ line haploid genome contains 100-200 V_H, 10-20 D, and 4 J_H elements. (Fig. 1B) Particular sequences (CACAGTC - spacer GCAAAAACC) are found next to V,D and J elements, differing for the lenght of the spacer (11 or 22 nucleotides).
These consensus sequences are thought to signal and mediate the rearrangements of the genetic elements which will form a variable gene (reviewed in 3).
It has been recently demonstrated that Ig genes rearrange "stepwise" during B cell ontogeny. The first molecular event recognizable in certain very immature pre B cells is a D-J_H rearrangement, which is followed by the rearrangement of a V_H gene to the preformed DJ_H - $C\mu$ complex.
As we shall see later, the VDJ-$C\mu$ complex can be actively transcribed and translated into a μ heavy chain. Only after an heavy chain gene has been successfully rearranged (it is obvious that this process is error -prone, and may easily result in "abortive" rearrangements producing frameshifts, stop codons etc), pre B cells proceed to rearrange L chain genes. It has been elegantly shown that K precede λ chain rearrangements. When an L chain has been successfully rearranged, H_2L_2 molecules can be formed and expressed on the cell surface by B lymphocytes (4).
The regulation of the genetic rearrangements of Ig genes is still obscure. It has been proposed that synthesis of μ chain inhibits further rearrangements at the IgH locus, concomitantly stimulating rearrangements of IgK and, if the rearrangement of K is unsuccessful, of the Igλ locus. The formation of an assembled H_2L_2 molecule may represent the signal to stop any further genetic rearrangement (with the exception of the isotype switch recombination, see below).

4) The generation of diversity of Ig molecules.

Ig diversity can be generated by recombinatorial mechanisms which assemble somatically a limited number of germ line encoded genes into an almost unlimited number of configurations. The minimum number of possible heavy chain variable regions is given by the number of V_H × the number of D × the number of J_H genes. This figure is further increased by several mechanisms. First, the D-J_H joining, as well as the V_L-J_L joining events, are "imprecise" with a variability which may extend over 10 nucleotides. Second, it has been shown that nucleotides may be inserted at the joining regions by the enzyme Terminal desoxynucleotide Transferase (TdT) which is very abundant in pre B cells. The junctional flexibility of V genes increases by at least an order of magnitude the number of V_H and V_L genes that can be created by somatic recombination (10^5 and 10^4 respectively are reasonable extimates). As the antigen binding site of an antibody molecule is formed by V_H and V_L sequences, we can create $\geqslant 10^9$ Ig variable regions ($V_H \times V_L$) with as few as 500 genetic elements. In addition, there is now ample evidence that Ig variable genes undergo somatic mutations at much higher rates than unrelated genes (e. g. C_H genes) (3).

5) <u>A second type of somatic recombination mediates isotype switching</u>

It is well known that IgM antibodies, predominating in the primary immune response, are replaced by IgG and IgA molecules of identical antigenic specificity in the course of the secondary response. This phenomenon, termed isotype switch, is mediated by a second type of somatic recombination (S-S recombination). A B cell clone first transcribes the VDJ-Cμ complex, which encodes a μ chain. Following "S-S" recombination there is the deletion of all the DNA comprised between the Sμ region and the S region of the C_H gene to be expressed. (e.g. γ1) The latter will replace the Cμ gene at the 3' end of the VDJ complex; in this configuration a γ_1 chain with identical variable region will be produced. Clusters of repetitive sequences (S regions) located at the left (5') of each C_H gene, mediate SS recombination (5). (See Fig. 2).

FIG. 2

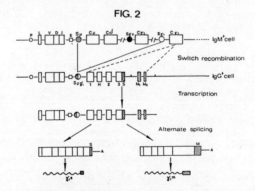

FIGURE 2.The mechanisms for isotype switching and for the synthesis of two
polypeptides differing at the COOH-termini(membrane bound and secreted heavy chains;the former have an hydrophobic C-terminal pep-
tide,which anchors the receptor molecule to the lipid bilayer,while
the latter have an hydrophilic C-terminus.)
The small circle indicates the promoter,the box(E)the enhancer, and
the bigger circles the switch regions. Big boxes indicate exons.

6) <u>The control of Ig expression</u>.

Although each of the many V_H and V_L genes is provided of promoter sequences in the 5' flanking regions, they are not expressed by non B cells. Furthermore, a given B cell transcribes only the V_H and V_L genes that have been rearranged. Thus, as originally

proposed by Tonegawa, V-C recombination activates Ig expression.
In 1983 the molecular basis of this phenomenon has been elucida-
ted: between J_L and C_L (in the case of heavy chains between J_H
and S_μ) are located the "enhancer" sequences. (6)
These sequences are indeed similar to the well known viral enhan-
cers, but differ from them for the property of being tissue-spe-
cific. Gene transfection experiments have shown that the Ig enhancer can increase the transcription of Ig genes in B lymphocytes, but not in fibroblasts. The enhancer acts on promoters
that can be located up to 10 kb apart in either directions (5'
or 3'). In the germ line configuration, the enhancer is too far
from the V genes to stimulate their transcription. After V-C
rearrangement, the enhancer is brought at $\sim$ 5-8 kb from the
promoter of the rearranged V gene, and can thus activate its
expression.

B) Chromosomal translocation involving immunoglobulin genes are
present in many lymphoproliferative disorders of the B cell
lineage.

1) Burkitt lymphomas

In 1972, Manolov and Manolova (7) reported that the vast majority ($\sim$ 80%) of Burkitt lymphomas (BL, a lymphoproliferative disorder of B lymphocytes particularly frequent in west
african children and related to the Epstein Barr Virus) display an 8:14 reciprocal translocation. Two other types of
translocations, 2:8 and 8:22 were later observed in the remaining cases ($\sim$ 15% and $\sim$ 5%, respectively).
These observation were followed with enormous interest, as
parallel studies had shown that Ig genes are located on chromosomes 14 (IgH), 2 (IgK) and 22 (Igλ). Further investigations revealed that in the case of the 8:14 (q24:q32) translocation, the breakpoint of chromosome 14 occurred actually
within the IgH locus (mapping at 14 q 32). Similarly, the
IgK (2p12) and the Igλ (22q11) loci were the targets of the
less frequent BL translocations. (8)

2) Murine myelomas

These results obtained on BLs were matched by studies in the
mouse, demonstrating frequent 15:12 or 15:6 translocations
in myelomas. In the mouse chromosome 12 harbors the IgH locus,
While IgK maps on chromosome 6. (9) Thus, compelling evidence
demonstrated that the immunoglobulin genes are directly involved in the translocations occurring in certain B cell malignancies. What about band q24 of human chromosome 8, which
is constantly involved in BL translocations, and band D 2/3 of
mouse chromosome 15 which rearrange in murine myelomas?

3) The translocations in BLs and murine myelomas involve Ig genes and the protooncogene cmyc.

Many laboratories have provided unequivocal evidence that in

both BL   and murine myelomas the gene involved in the translocation encodes the protooncogene c-myc (10-14). Protooncogenes
(c-onc) are a family of genes which are found in the normal genome of all species and are homologous to viral genes (v-onc)
found in tumorigenic retroviruses (8,10). Malignant transformation of susceptible cells may be induced by either retrovirus
infection or, more importantly, by introducing in the cell
(transfection) isolated genes, purified by means of recombinant
DNA technology. These results demonstrate that specific genes
(oncogenes) may be responsible for establishing the transformed
phenotype. These genes, originally found in RNA viruses (v-onc)
have their counterpart within normal cells (c-onc). Although
structural differences may be found between v-onc and c-onc, it
is generally accepted that they encode identical proteins, and
that such proteins play a fundamental role in regulating cellular
growth.
In the normal cell, protooncogenes are subjected to a rigorous
control of their expression. Alterations of this strict control
may result in the malignant transformation. Mechanisms of deregulation of c-onc expression include structural changes within
the coding sequences (a "ras" gene with a point mutation leading
to a gly → val substitution at position 12, has been isolated
from a bladder carcinoma but not from its normal counterpart),
or within the regulatory elements flanking the c-onc. For in-
stance, insertion of a promoter elements of viral origin may
follow infection with "slow" retroviruses, that is viruses lacking v-onc but carrying LTR sequences. If the insertion occurs
in the vicinity of c-onc genes it may result in malignant
transformation.
In addition, v-onc are in the viral genome in close proximity to
certain sequences termed long terminal repeats (LTR) which act
as strong promoter/enhancer. Viral infection (or integration
of the virus in the cellular genome) will result in over expression of the v-onc gene(s).
In the case of BLs and murine myelomas the knowledge of the
structure of Ig genes immediately led to the proposal that the
chromosomal translocations brought the c-myc gene under the
control of the Ig regulatory elements, which are very active in
B cells. The properties of the Ig enhancer, bidirectional long
distance activity, made it a good candidate for the deregulation
of c-myc which occurs in BLs and murine myelomas.
Extensive sequence analysis of the chromosomal breakpoints demonstrated that if in the case of the BL cell line "Manca" the
enhancer model was correct, in the case of other BL cell lines
(e.g. RAMOS) the 8:14 caused a deletion of the Ig enhancer.(Fig.3).
Other mechanisms, such as alterations in the chromatine structure,
somatic mutations or translational deregulation of the translo-
cated c-myc may be invoked in these cases (8-14).

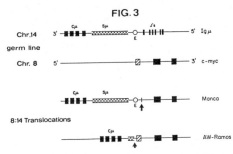

FIGURE 3.Analysis of the 8:14 chromosomal breakpoints(indicated
by arrows) in two Burkitt Lymphoma cell lines(Manca and
AW-Ramos). Note that the transcriptional orientation of
the μ and c-myc genes is opposite:the two genes rearrange"head to head". In the case of Manca the translocation
has brought the two coding exons of c-myc(black boxes)
next to the Ig enhancer(open circle),while in AW-Ramos
the enhancer has been deleted,and the first(non-coding)
exon(hatched box) is still in his germ line configura-
tion.Adapted from ref.10.

4) Chronic lymphocytic leukemias and non-Burkitt B cell
lymphomas.

A recent series of studies, conducted in the laboratory of
Carlo Croce in Philadelphia (15), demonstrated two new types
of translocations in certain human chronic lymphocytic leukemias and B lymphomas. (14:11 and 14:18). Again, translocations involving IgH genes are detected in B cell malignancies. Analysis of the breakpoints of each translocations
revealed the existence of two new putative oncogenes, bcl.1
and bcl.2. No viral homologs have been found yet for bcl.1
and bcl.2. A striking observation is however that bcl.1
and bcl.2 genes are flanked by the same heptamer-spacer-
nonamer sequences which mediate VDJ recombinations.
A parallel survey of T cell malignancies has revealed a series of translocations which involve putative oncogenes (tcl.
1; tcl.2) and the genes encoding the antigen receptor of T
cells, which rearrange somatically in a manner similar to
immunoglobulin genes.
The interaction between somatic cell genetics and molecular
genetics is thus opening the way to define not only new
oncogenes, but possibly also new rearranging gene families.

C) The I.29 B cell lymphoma: an in vitro a model for the study of
B cell differentiation.

Tumor cell lines may be considered the clonal expansion of a
cell at a given stage of differentiation. Much of the work on
Ig genes has been conducted on myelomas, the malignant counter-

part of plasmacells. The latter are cells devoled to Ig secretion, and represent the terminal stage of B cell differentiation. If an impressive amount of knowledge has accumulated on the rearrangements of Ig genes, the sequences mediating these rearrangements etc., rather little is known on the regulation of these events in the course of B cell differentiation.

To gain information about this, one should have a panel of cell lines capable of differentiation in vitro.

In our laboratory we have studied extensively one such cell line, the murine lymphoma I.29 (16) I.29 is a monoclonal (as defined by the idiotypic specificities of Ig molecules) B cell lymphoma, expressing membrane associated IgM. Stimulation of I.29 μ^+ cells in vitro with B cell mitogens such as lipopolysaccharide (LPS) (17) induces two differentiative events: the majority ($\sim$80%) of the cells differentiate into IgM secreting plasmacells, while variable proportions of cells (5-10%) switch to α or ε production. (18-19) The two differentiative pathways are mutually exclusive, as differentiation into μ^+ plasmacells leads to a drastic arrest in proliferation, while switch to α or ε implies deletion of the expressed μ gene (as well as all the other C_H genes located 5' to the one that will be expressed).

Plasmacell differentiation is characterized by several changes in Ig biosynthesis: first of all there is an absolute increase in the rate of transcription of the VDJ-Cμ complex. In addition there is a drastic change in the splicing pattern of the Cμ 3' terminus, with an unbalance in favor μ_S encoding transcripts over μ_m mRNAs (see lower part of fig. 2). The μ_S mRNA increases 8-15 folds. At the protein level, μ_S chain biosynthesis increases in parallel, while μ_m chains are no longer synthesized.

This is in contrast with an actual increase (1.5-2 folds) of the μ_m mRNA. Taken together these data indicate that the μ_m mRNA is translationally regulated in the differentiating μ^+ cell, and raise the question of how this regulation may act, as the 2 transcripts, μ_m and μ_S, are identical for more than 1700 nucleotides at the 5' end.(20) Interestingly, the regulation of α_m- α_S and $\varepsilon_m/\varepsilon_S$ chains, analyzed in identical experiments conducted on α^+ and ε^+ I.29 cells, is regulated at the pretranslational level (21-22). The reasons for this difference between μ and other isotypes, and the biological role of the increased μ_m mRNA (no longer translated) in differentiating μ^+ cells are obscure.

In line with other tumor cell line systems, induction of differentiation is matched by an arrest in cell proliferation (17). We have analyzed c-myc transcription in several I.29 derived cell lines; in all these cell lines there are no detectable rearrangements of c-myc, which is however transcribed abundantly. LPS stimulation of μ^+, α^+ or ε^+ cells is followed by a decrease in c-myc transcription. We are currently investigating rearrangements and transcription of other oncogenes in I.29 cells.

The I.29 tumor is an optimal model for studying isotype switching, as we have the possibility of analyzing both the precursor and the switched cells.

An analysis of several α^+ clones has demonstrated that SS recombination occurs in different points of the S_α regions in different clones. Moreover the sequence of the variable gene is <u>identical</u> in μ^+ and α^+ cells, indicating that in the case of I.29, isotype switching is not accompanied by somatic mutations in the VDJ complex (Klein and Stavnezer, in preparation). Rearrangements and deletions have been demonstrated also on the "excluded" chromosome (that is the chromosome in which no VDJ recombination has taken place): the extent of the deletions on the excluded chromosome vary from clone to clone (18), implying that the hypothetical "switch recombinases" that mediate   recombination may act "in trans".
We have recently addressed the question of whether a single μ^+ cell can undergo both isotype switching and plasmacell differentiation, or whether distinct "precommitted" precursors exist in the I.29 lymphoma. To this end we have cloned I.29 μ^+ cells and analyzed individual clones for their differentiative potentials. 100% of the clones are able to differentiate into μ^+ plasmacells while only a proportion of them (73%) can undergo isotype switching in response to LPS. Interestingly, there seems to be a pre-committment to switch to either $\mathcal{E}$ or α in individual clones (23) The reasons for such precommittment, certainly operating in a negative sense in respect to C_γ genes (never expressed by I.29 cells) may involve the structure of chromatine (19), the existence of class specific "switch recombinases etc.

Although the bias of working with a "transformed" cell line should be always kept in mind, the I.29 system could offer the answer to several problems dealing with the regulatory mechanisms of B cell differentiation.

Acknowledgements

I am indebted with Drs. C. Alberini,S.De Ambrosis, A.Rubartelli, G.Vidali and D.Vismara for many stimulating discussion, with Drs. D.Klein and J.Stavnezer for communicating results before publication, and to Ms. G.Tirelli for typing the manuscript. This work was in part supported by a grant from Consiglio Nazionale Ricerche, Progetto Finalizzato Ingegneria Genetica.

REFERENCES

1) Jeske D. and Capra J.D. (1984) In Fundamental Immunology. Paul W E editor. Raven Press p. 131.

2) Hozumi N. and Tonegawa S. (1976) Proc.Natl.Acad.Sci USA 73:3628.

3) Tonegawa S. (1983) Nature 302:575

4) Korsmeyer S.J., Hieter P.A., Ravetch J.V., Poplack D.G., Waldmann T.A., and Leder P. (1981) Proc.Natl.Acad.Sci. USA 78:7096.

5) Yaoita Y. and Honjo T. (1980) Nature 286:650.

6) Gillies et al. (1983) Cell 33:717; Banerji et al. (1983) Cell 33:729; Queen and Baltimore (1983) Cell 33:341.

7) Manolov G. and Manolova Y. 1972 Nature 237:33.

8) Klein G. (1981) Nature 294:313; Klein G. (1983) Cell 32:311; Perry R.P. (1983) Cell 33:647.

9) Stanton L.W. et al. (1983) Nature 303:401; Gerondakis et al. (1984) Cell 36:973.

10) Oncogenes and Viral Genes. (1984) Vander Woulde G.F., Levine A.J., Topp W.C. and Watson J.D. editors. CSH Laboratory publisher;

11) Rushdi A.A., Nishikura K., Erikson J., Watt R., Rovera G. and Croce C.M. (1983) Science 222:390.

12) Rabbitts T.H., Hamlyn P.H. and Baer R. (1983). Nature 306:760.

13) Taub R., Moulding C., Battey J., Murphy W., Vasicek T., Lenok G.M. and Leder P. (1984) Cell 36:339.

14) Hayday A.C., Gillies S.D., Saito H., Wood C., Wiman K., Hayward W.S. and Tonegawa S. (1984) Nature 307:334.

15) Croce C.M. et al. (1985) in press.

16) Sitia R., Rubartelli A. and Hammerling U. (1981) J.Immunol. 127:1388.

17) Sitia R., Rubartelli A., DeAmbrosis S., Pozzi D. and Hammerling U. (1985) Eur. J. Immunol. in press.

18) Stavnezer J., Sirlin S. and Abbott J. (1985) J.Exp.Med. 161:577.

19) Stavnezer J., Abbott J. and Sirlin S. (1984) Curr. Top. Microbiol. Immunol. 113:109.

20) Sitia R., Alberini C., DeAmbrosis S., Rubartelli A. and Hammerling U. (1985) Manuscript submitted.

21) Sitia R., Rubartelli A., Kikutani H., Hammerling U. and Stavnezer J. (1985) J.Immunol. in press.

22) Sitia R. (1985) Molec. Immunol. in press.

23) Alberini C., DeAmbrosis S., Vismara D. and Sitia R. (1985) in preparation.

The Immune System and the Central Nervous System: Separation or Communication?

G. Tridente

Institute of Immunological Sciences, University of Verona,
Verona, Italy

ABSTRACT

The author presents a critical analysis of data and opinions in the recent literature concerning interaction between the CNS and the IS via anatomical and molecular mediators. The overall picture is that of two highly complex, interacting compartments with bidirectional stimulatory and inhibitory feedback. The IS shows particular microenvironmental adaptation in the brain, which allows antigen presentation and recognition via the endothelial astrocyte system and more limited expression of the effector phase of immune reactivity. Neuro-inducers and immune molecules flow freely in the two systems, and a considerable sharing of antigens and receptors is documented. It is concluded that both separation and communication occur between the CNS and the IS, guaranteeing reciprocal protection of the different microenvironments and homeostatic regulation.

KEYWORDS

Immune system; central nervous system; networks; neuro-immunoregulation.

INTRODUCTION

In his initial impact with the central nervous system (CNS) the immunologist comes up against a barrier (Leibowitz and Hughes, 1983). In fact, the brain is isolated from the general immune system (IS); it lacks organized lymphoid tissue and lymphatic drainage, and is cut off from the circulation by a selective blood-brain barrier which prevents the entry of large molecules, such as many antigens and antibodies. Therefore, CNS immune defense is only possible from the outside, while in all other body sites, with a few minor exceptions, lymphoid detectors and effectors can flow freely and act in situ. As a consequence, intracerebral antigens, whether endogenous or accidental, escape immune recognition. On the other hand, when the selective barrier is somehow eluded or interrupted, the CNS is rapidly transformed into a complex and unusual battlefield, where all sorts of immunopathologic lesions can be detected, with unique expressions determined by the way the specialized tissues of the brain respond to antigenic and immunologic injury.

This context apparently excludes any physiological role of the IS within the CNS, which seems only to suffer from immunopathologic attacks when the crucial function of the blood-brain barrier is impaired. It is evident that such a situation appears unique as well as highly unstable and fragile to the immuno- logist. In fact, modern immunology has revealed the existence of multiple fine molecular mechanisms for controlling the immune response, showing that both potentiating and auppressive regulatory networks are constantly operating in the modulation of immune reactivity in order to keep the effector mechanisms within physiological limits (Jerne, 1974; Moeller, 1984). A crucial factor in such physiological dimensioning is the presence of different receptors on the surface of lymphocytes (Moretta et al, 1982) which allow cell-to-cell interactions, specific antigen recognition, and genetically controlled restric- tions (Accolla et al, 1984) of the immune response. A second crucial event is the discrimination for "self-determinants" (Grossman, 1984), which implies direct 'education' of lymphocytes on autoantigens. Such multi-controlled, dynamic operativity of the IS is safer and more stable when continuous confront- ation with autoantigens is possible. Therefore, obsolete 'sequestered' antigen- ic sites are potentially dangerous and unlikely to be extensively present in the body. Absolute sequestration of autoantigens has been suspected in various other organs (thyroid, testicles, etc.), and the loss of such isolation has been indicated as a critical factor in the pathogenesis of autoimmune reactions (Holborow, 1981). In fact, most of these 'sanctuaries' have been shown not to be true sequestered sites, and the respective autoimmune aggres- sions are now considered as the pathologic expression of physiological auto- immune recognitions, due to an imbalance of immunoregulatory (suppressive) mechanisms and antigenic cross-reactions (Kunkel, 1983; Waksman, 1984).

On this basis, the dogmatic concept of absolute separation for the whole CNS appears highly improbable in the eyes of immunologists. In fact, most of the recent evidence points to the existence of immune circuits and responses in the CNS, which, however, operate within certain constraints. The immunoglobulin level in the cerebrospinal fluid (CSF) is low but not absent. The CSF/serum ratio is 1:100 and that of IgG is approximately 1:300; however, in fetal CSF the concentration of IgG (maternal) rises to 160 mg/l. Moreover, in some cere- bral districts, such as the area postrema, the tuber cinereum and the posterior pituitary, proteins easily enter from the blood stream, as evidenced by the Evans blue dye test. The number of lymphocytes within the CNS is low, but rapidly increases during inflammatory, autoimmune and neoplastic processes (Leibowitz and Hughes, 1983). Recent data, mainly derived from tumor grafting experiments, indicate the existence of immune effector mechanisms within the CNS (Forni et al, 1984; Saris et al, 1984), although these are reduced by recognition of intracerebral antigens and, possibly, by the production of high-molecular-weight inhibiting factors (Schwyzer and Fontana, 1985). Thus, it seems more likely that classic immune responses are not compatible with the highly interactive nervous network; therefore, particular forms of immune defense and communication may have developed between the two major systems as a consequence of mutual adaptation. If this approach is correct, one may find signs of:
- intercommunication between the CNS and the IS;
- particular immune microenvironments within the CNS.
In fact, consistent experimental support is accumulating   in favor of this

hypothesis, and in particular:
- the CNS produces a number of effects on the IS, i.e. the two systems communicate in both directions;
- there is a remarkable presence of 'immune' molecules within the CNS, i.e. a particular 'microimmune' internal network can be postulated;
- there is a counterpart of 'nervous' molecules and receptors on cells of the immune system, i.e. in both sites there are molecules and receptors for mutual communication;
- there is extensive sharing of molecules and receptors by the CNS and the IS.

Under these circumstances the blood-brain-barrier should be interpreted as the necessary separation of two different microenvironmental compartments with differently adapted defense mechanisms, rather than as an impenetrable diaphragm preventing communication between the CNS and the IS.

CNS CONTROL OVER THE IMMUNE SYSTEM

Neurophysiological and immunological approaches have been applied to the analysis of the intricate connections between the CNS and IS. Such links are anatomical and functional, as revealed by different experimental models, including innervation studies of lymphoid organs, Pavlovian conditioning and localized destruction of CNS areas (Table 1). More recent data have enriched our knowledge of neurotransmitters and neuroendocrine molecules affecting the IS. Therefore, the foundations have been laid for new interdisciplinary fields such as neuroimmunology, neuroimmunomodulation and, to the more enthusiastic minds, psychoimmunology (Ader, 1981; Fabris et al, 1983).

Particular attention has been devoted to the thymus, which is considered the crucial differentiator and regulator of immune reactivity (Tridente, 1985). The autonomic innervation of the thymus has long been known; more recently, thymic innervation has been traced back to ventral spinal horns, to the retrofacial nucleus and to the nucleus ambiguus (Bullock and Moore, 1981). The human fetal thymus is innervated starting from the eleventh week of gestation; innervation not only reaches the capsule and the vessels, but deepens in the cortex and the medulla in close proximity to differentiating thymocytes. Both in rodents and in humans bearing immune defects or thymic abnormalities, the innervation was found to be aberrant (Ghali et al, 1980). Other primary (bone marrow, bursa of Fabricius) and secondary (spleen, lymph nodes) lymphoid organs have complex innervations, suggesting more delicate neural influences on the parenchyma, other than simple vascular control (Spector, 1983; Felten et al, 1985). Pavlovian conditioning has been used to induce suppression of antibody production, of delayed-type hypersensitivity and graft-vs-host reactions (Ader, 1981, 1983), as well as an increase in natural killer (NK) cells (Ghanta et al, 1985). Such influences involve stress conditioning and susceptibility to infectious and neoplastic diseases, possibly via hypothalamic intervention (Stein et al, 1976).

Interesting results have been obtained by electrolytic, chemical and physical destruction of particular CNS areas (Cross et al, 1980; Forni et al, 1983, 1984; Roszman et al, 1985), mainly of the hypothalamus and neocortex. Damage to the former produces a reduction in number and function of T and NK cells; neocortical lesions (mainly of the left hemisphere) similarly impair both compartments (Renoux, 1984).

Table 1. Central Nervous System effects on the Immune System.

Action	Effect
Pavlovian conditioning	Suppression of Ab production and DTH, increased NK activity
CNS lesions:	
- electrolytic and chemical	Reduced T and NK function/number
- asymmetric (neocortex)	Left: reduced T function/number
	Right: increased T function/number
Neuroendocrine mediators:	
a) Via innervation	
- norepinephrine	Positive/negative immunoregulation
- serotonin	Positive/negative immunoregulation
- acetylcholine	Lymphocyte proliferation
b) Via pituitary peptides (lymphokine effect)	
- ACTH	In vitro suppression of Ab response
- opiate endorphins	Immunosuppression, macrophage chemotaxis, increased tumorigenicity (effects blocked by naloxone)
- growth hormone (GH)	In vitro generation of CTL, impairment of DTH in GH deficiency
- ARG-vasopressin, oxytocin, bombesin, enkephalins	IL-2 effect on T cells (γ-IFN), macrophage chemotaxis
- thyrotropin	In vitro enhancement of Ab response
- substance P, neurotensin	Increased T-cell mitogenesis, degranulation of mast cells, macrophage chemotaxis
- somatostatin	Inhibition of anti-SRBC Ab production, blocking of mast cells (leukotrienes)

More precise information was produced by analysis of the effects of neuroendocrine mediators on the IS. In fact, many molecules have been shown to induce positive and negative immunoregulatory effects as summarized in Table 1. The overall picture clearly points to inducible effects on the IS at different levels. Serotonin and catecholamines reduce the primary IgM and IgG antibody response and decrease the immunologic memory and the mitogenic (PHA, ConA) response, while enhancing the production of corticosteroids (Crary et al, 1983; Rosman et al, 1985).

Acetylcholine has been shown to interfere with the proliferation of thymocytes (Tridente et al, 1978; Singh, 1979); the existence of specific receptors on thymocytes (Fuchs et al, 1980; Pizzighella et al, 1982; Riviera et al, 1985), thymic epithelial cells (Engel et al, 1977) and thymus extracts (Raimond et al, 1984) has been repeatedly demonstrated.

The effect of enkephalins–endorphins on various functions of the immune system has recently been reviewed (Plotnikoff and Murso, 1985), showing distinct effects on antibody synthesis, lymphocyte proliferation and NK activity (Mathews et al, 1983; Wybran, 1985). These effects, like those mediated by ACTH, have been compared to the effect of lymphokines on the immune system and are also shared by other hormones and pituitary peptides. Growth hormone (GH) is under the control of a releasing factor (GRF) of hypothalamic origin (Bloch et al, 1983; Spiess et al, 1983) and induces the generation of cytotoxic lymphocytes (CTL) in vitro (Snow et al, 1981). Vasopressin, oxytocin, substance P, neurotensin and other peptides have complex effects on the IS, including stimulatory effects mimicking or replacing the effects of IL-2 (Johnson and Torres, 1985). They also increase T-cell mitogenesis and induce macrophage chemotaxis and degranulation of mast cells. On the contrary, somatostatin has inhibiting effects on antibody production and on the release of leukotrienes from mastocytes (Goetzl et al, 1985).

Taken together, these data definitely indicate that the CNS has a number of efferent limbs to communicate with, and influence, immune functions. T cells, B cells, macrophages and NK cells all receive inhibitory or stimulatory signals, thus proving the existence of neuro–immunoregulatory circuits. It may be postulated, therefore, that the IS sends back signals to the CNS and that both systems possess similar receptors to receive signals from both neuromolecules and immunomolecules.

THE IMMUNE CONTROL SYSTEM OF THE BRAIN

By analogy with other types of regulatory mechanisms a reciprocal flow of information is essential to generate homeostatic regulatory control. Therefore, an afferent limb to the CNS from the IS is to be expected. Two major aspects of immuno–neuro communication have recently been identified: the pattern of signalling from the general immune system to the CNS and the microimmune network acting within the CNS.

a) Immune signals to the CNS

Table 2 summarizes a number of immune functions and molecules which produce neuroendocrine effects. An antibody response to sheep red cells or TNP hemocyanin increases the neuronal firing rate in the rat hypothalamus (Besedovsky et al, 1983a); the peak of the antibody response correlates with the peak of neuronal firing and with a marked decrease in catecholamines in the hypothalamus, but not in other brain areas (Besedovsky et al, 1983c). The situation also gives rise to an increase in glucocorticoids. Therefore, the circuitry would appear to send information to the CNS regarding the generation of an immune response at the periphery, which, in turn, generates modulatory countersignals via catecholamines and glucocorticoids (Besedovsky et al, 1983b).

Table 2. Neuro-immune Intercommunication.

Action	Effect
Primary immune response	- increased neuronal firing rate (hypothalamus) - increased glucocorticoids
Lymphocyte soluble factors (mitogen-induced)	- increased corticosterone (ACTH-mediated?)
Thymosin	- increased ACTH, glucocorticoids and beta- endorphin
Interleukin-1 (IL-1)	- induction of slow-wave sleep - endogenous CNS production
Interleukin-2 (IL-2)	- increased ACTH and cortisol
Interferon	- slow-wave sleep, lethargy, fever

Similar effects are generated by lymphocyte soluble factors released in culture and, more specifically, by interleukins (IL-1 and IL-2), interferon and thymic hormones (Hall and Goldstein, 1983), which are present in supernatants of mitogen-stimulated lymphocyte cultures. Thymosin (fraction 5), injected into monkeys, elevates corticotropin, beta-endorphin and cortisol, while thymectomy exerts opposite effects (Healy et al, 1983). Thymosins and lymphokines can stimulate the pituitary-adrenal axis; evidence has been produced to show that they act on the CNS and can also be produced in situ. However, these factors are devoid of direct effects on the adrenal cortex (Hall et al, 1985b). It is worth mentioning that, in addition to other immune and neuroendocrine effects, IL-1 and interferon produce central effects such as slow-wave sleep, depression, lethargy and fever (Krueger et al, 1984; Abrams et al, 1985). Therefore, a counterpart of the 'neurotransmitters' which flow from the CNS to the IS does exist, and the term 'immunotransmitters' has been proposed for them (Hall et al, 1985a).

b) The intracerebral microimmune network

One of the important assumptions regarding the inability of the IS to operate within the CNS is based on the difficulty of detecting molecules and cells pertaining to the former system in the context of nervous tissue. However, immune responses do take place in the CNS, albeit with limitations. In fact, in normal tissue, lymphocytes and antibodies are poorly represented and macrophages are virtually absent, but infections and neoplastic processes induce a rapid input of all sorts of immune effectors. Therefore, the CNS, although separated from the general immune system and behaving in part as an immunologically privileged site, may possess particular immune circuits capable of recognizing internal antigens in order to regulate intracerebral responses and possibly send signals to the outer part of the IS. It is expected that such recognition mechanisms, though mediated by immunological molecules, should somehow differ from the conventional macrophage-mediated antigen presentation, because of the specialized microenvironment in which they operate.

Antigen recognition needs presentation to T helper cells by accessory cells displaying class II (DR) glycoproteins (Accolla et al, 1984) of the major histocompatibility complex (MHC), which have to be corecognized along with the antigen by antigen-specific T cells. Macrophages and different kinds of dendritic cells (all identified as accessory cells) share this property and are rich in DR molecules, and some produce an interleukin (IL-1) which acts as an essential second activating signal for T helper cells. The latter, when activated, produce IL-2 acting as a clonal T expander of various effector lymphocyte subsets (Roitt et al, 1985). DR expression can be induced by a number of factors, such as mitogens and interferon, or inhibited by prostaglandin E and alpha-fetoprotein. Therefore, DR molecules and IL-1 are considered as essential factors for antigen recognition and the subsequent modulation of the immune response (Janeway et al, 1984).

In the CNS these molecules have recently been traced (Fontana et al, 1983; de Tribolet et al, 1984a), and the vascular endothelium and astrocytes have been proposed as specialized accessory cells; these cells are thought to act as a bidirectional interconnecting system between the brain and the general IS (Fontana and Fierz, 1985). In fact, endothelial cells are in direct contact with the blood stream and express class II antigens (Hayry et al, 1980), mainly after induction by activated T cells and by gamma-interferon (Pober et al, 1983). Astrocytes are in direct contact both with endothelial cells and neuronal surfaces (White et al, 1981; Kimelbers et al, 1983) via their cytoplasmic processes (Hayry et al, 1980). Moreover, astrocytes show modulation of surface class II antigens (Wong et al, 1984) and active production of IL-1 (Fontana and Fierz, 1985). The latter is active on T lymphocytes and appears to be very similar to macrophage IL-1 (Dinarello, 1984). Recently, the presentation of the myelin basic protein antigen by astrocytes to T lymphocytes has been demonstrated in the rat (Fontana et al, 1984).

In conclusion, the chain of molecular transmitters for antigen recognition and induction of immune signals seems to be fully present within the CNS, though mediated by different specialized 'accessory' cells. The limited expression of immune reactivity in the CNS, therefore, cannot be ascribed simply to the presence of the blood-brain barrier or to the scarcity of antigen-presenting cells, but may be due to multi-regulatory molecular effects restricted to such a specialized microenvironment. In this context it is important to note that glioblastoma cells produce prostaglandin E (DR inhibitor) and release a 95000 mol. wt. factor in culture which inhibits the effect of IL-1 (Fontana et al, 1982, 1984).

SHARED MOLECULES AND RECEPTORS

Although separated by anatomical and functional devices, the CNS microenvironment communicates with the general IS and/or with the internal specialized immunoenvironment. Therefore, part of the molecules and receptors of both systems have to be shared in order to code and decode bidirectional signals. Indeed, a number of structural homologies and functional effects have been detected between immune and neural compartments. Table 3 lists a number of 'immune' molecules which are present in the brain. The Thy-1 antigen is particularly interesting since it is present in mouse thymocytes and in human thymic epithelial cells as well as in neuronal cells (Williams and Gagnon, 1982). Mouse brain Thy-1 glycoprotein presents a good structural homology with immunoglobulin domains (mainly with the variable domain) and with beta$_2$-microglobulin (a constituent of class-I MHC antigens). In the rat, the monoclonal antibody MRC OX2 recognizes antigens present in thymocytes, brain cells, vascular endothelial cells and other types of cells (Barclay and Ward, 1982). Human brain and fibroblasts contain Thy-1 homologues which are structurally and antigenically related (but not identical) to rodent Thy-1 (Cotmore et al, 1981). Thy-1 analogues are present even in invertebrates (squid), which suggests that this glycoprotein may represent a primordial immunoglobulin and an important receptor for cell interactions (Williams, 1982). An important indication comes from experiments on chickens in which a species-specific anti-Thy-1 antibody inhibits the formation of long-term memory (Bernard et al., 1983). Other molecules not necessarily related to the immunoglobulin superfamily, such as the rat W3/13 antigen, are shared by the thymus and the brain (Brown et al, 1981). Finally, the endogenous synthesis of IL-1 in macrophages and astrocytes and their complex actions on the IS (T helper cell activation) and CNS (sleep, fever) have been previously mentioned.

Table 3. Presence of 'Immune' Molecules within the Central Nervous System.

Antigen	Localization
Thy-1 (mouse, man)	- brain (neurons), thymus - anti-Thy-1 antibodies inhibit long-term memory
OX2 (rat)	- brain (homogenate), thymus, dendritic cells, etc.
MHC class II	- brain (astrocytes), glioma (modulation by γ-IFN)
MHC class I	- enhancement in astrocytes, oligodendrocytes, microglia and some neurons by γ-IFN
T8 (man)	- oligodendrocytes (ovine), T suppressor/cytotoxic
W3/13 (rat)	- brain, thymus, leukocytes
IL-1	- brain (endogenous synthesis), macrophages

On the other hand, a number of neuroinducers (peptides, hormones, transmitters), mainly related to hypothalamic function, interact with cellular components of the IS (Table 4). For most of these substances specific receptors have been postulated or identified on lymphocytes, thymocytes and mast cells (Payan and Goetzl, 1985; O'Dorisio et al, 1985; Goetzl et al, 1985). Moreover, some of the most typical neuropeptides and hormones, such as ACTH and endorphins, are also synthesized in vitro by lymphocytes after polyclonal mitogen stimulation or virus infection (Smith and Blalock, 1981); other hormones which undergo hypothalamic control have been found in human leukocytes and mouse spleen cells (Blalock et al, 1985). These data indicate not only that the IS may be influenced by CNS products, but that some of them may also be synthesized within the IS and act as immune auto-regulators; however, it cannot be ruled out that such extracerebral products may also influence the nervous and the endocrine system.

Table 4.   Presence of Nervous Molecules in the Immune System.

Molecules	Cells
Receptors:	
Neuropeptides	Lymphocytes, mast cells
Neurohormones	Lymphocytes
Neurotransmitters	Thymocytes
Cross-reacting antigens:	
Myelin-associated glycoprotein	NK cells
Glioma GE$_2$ antigen	Epithelial thymus

Occasional findings have revealed the existence of other antigenic structures, initially considered specific to the CNS compartment, which are shared by some important components of the IS. The monoclonal antibody HNK1 (Leu 7), which recognizes a membrane antigen of NK cells, has been found to bind to myelin and myelin-forming cells (Schuller-Petrovic et al, 1983). Subsequently, this antigen has been recognized as a myelin-associated glycoprotein (MAG), and the shared specificity refers to the epitope recognized by autoantibodies of patients suffering from demyelinating neuropathies (McGarry et al, 1983; Steck and Murray, 1985). A second occasional finding has revealed that an anti-Thy-1 monoclonal antibody also binds specifically to vimentin (Dulbecco et al, 1981). A third occasional finding is related to the well-known antiglioma antibody GE$_2$ (Schnegg et al, 1981). This antibody was occasionally found to be positive also in spleen, thymus and kidney cells (de Tribolet et al, 1984b). We have shown that GE$_2$ binds specifically to thymic cortical epithelial cells (Tridente et al, this volume), which constitute an important component related to the synthesis of thymic hormones (Haynes and Heisenbarth, 1983; Tridente, 1985).

LOOPS AND NETWORKS

The way all the products and cells involved in CNS-IS interaction may operate is

still difficult to understand. However, preliminary hypotheses have been
proposed with the aim of initiating the systematic analysis of mutual influences. Such models include essentially the hypothalamic-endocrine axis and the
thymus-lymphocyte axis as the two stem branches of embryogenetic, anatomical,
functional and molecular connections between the CNS and IS (Besedovsky et al,
1983a; Hall and Goldstein, 1983; Spector, 1983; Blalock and Smith, 1985; Hall et
al, 1985b; Smith et al, 1985). In these hypothetical schemes, adrenal, thyroid
and gonadal hormones are more directly involved as feedback regulators. Finally,
interesting hypotheses have also been proposed concerning neocortical parti-
cipation in the neuroendocrine networks, thus indicating new approaches for
behavioral and stress conditioning of immunological and neoplastic diseases
(Stein et al, 1976; Ader, 1981; Renoux, 1984; Ghanta et al, 1985; Marx, 1985;
Pert et al, 1985). Although preliminary, these indications present a stimulating
challenge for future investigations.

SEPARATION AND COMMUNICATION

It is premature to draw definitive conclusions on the basis of such intricate
and preliminary background information. However, a few basic questions may be
considered as sufficiently clarified at this time:

1) there is little doubt that the IS exerts a measure of control over the CNS
not only from the border, i.e. from outside the blood-brain barrier, but
directly from the inside. Such control is comprehensive of the very initial
steps of immune reactivity, i.e. antigen recognition. However, this task would
not appear to be performed by conventional macrophages, but by specialized cells
of the endothelial-astrocyte system (Fontana and Fierz, 1985). The latter cells
undoubtedly possess the basic requisites of antigen-presenting cells.

2) Immune molecules are sufficiently represented within the normal CNS and
rapidly increase during inflammatory and neoplastic states. The immune
reactivity, however, seems to be more restrained in the CNS than in other body
sites. Glial cells and glioblastoma cells have been shown to produce IL-1, but
also to synthesize an inhibitory protein which blocks the activatory signals of
the interleukin (Schwyzer and Fontana, 1984). Therefore, this immune microenvironment is peculiar to the CNS and can easily be further suppressed by endogenous neoplastic growth.

3) CNS control of, and communication with, the IS are supported by stronger
experimental evidence. The efferent limb is mainly governed by hypothalamic
structures and involves stimulatory and inhibitory signals transmitted directly
or via the endocrine system to the general IS (Fig. 1). Even neocortical and
psychic influences cannot be excluded, although it would appear to be somewhat
premature to attempt to explain such phenomena in psychoimmunological terms
(Maddox, 1984).

4) A number of molecules, which may be either 'nervous' or 'immune', are shared
by the CNS and the IS. The list is increasing and indicates more than occasional
cross-reactivities. Receptors for both groups are also shared. Finally, some IS
molecules are synthesized by CNS cells and vice versa. The integration seems
fully justified, even if it is not completely clear.

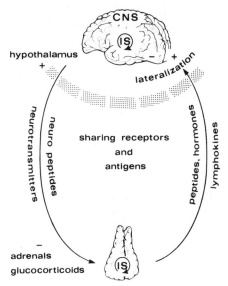

Fig. 1. The neuro-immune network.

Going back to the initial question as to whether there is separation or communication between the CNS and the IS and striking a balance between the most dogmatic (the privileged site, closed off by barriers) and the most enthusiastic positions (the IS as a sensory organ or mobile brain), it seems to us that there is enough proof of the existence of both separation and communication between the two systems. The separation is not absolute and it would seem more justifiable to postulate the existence of two different immune environments (the general IS and the intracerebral immune microenvironment) than to insist on absolute exclusion of immune control within the CNS. The case for communication between the two systems rests essentially on the homeostatic leadership of the CNS over all other regulatory networks, including the immune network. Moreover, the existence of two different immune environments (the general and the cerebral) which are sufficiently protected by anatomical partitions, but are fully interacting at molecular level, provides further evidence of communication.

ACKNOWLEDGEMENTS AND NOTES

This work was supported in part by the Italian National Research Council (C.N.R.) under the Oncology Research Project, by the Ministry of Education and by ARBI, Verona. The author wishes to thank Mrs. Liliana Pascoli for the drawings and Mr. Anthony Steele for editing the text of this paper.
In view of the interdisciplinary scope of the Meeting, the references selected for this paper were mainly general reviews.

REFERENCES

Abrams, P.G., E. McClamrock and K.A. Foon (1985). N. Engl. J. Med., 312, 443-445.
Accolla, R.S., A. Moretta and S. Carrel (1984). Sem. Hematol., 21, 287-295.

Ader, R. (1981). Psychoneuroimmunology, Academic Press, New York.

Ader, R. (1983). In: Immunoregulation, Plenum Press, New York, 283-313.

Barclay, A.N. and H.A. Ward (1982). Eur. J. Biochem., 129, 447-458.

Bernard, C.C.A., M.E. Gibbs, R.J. Hodge and K.J. Ng (1983). Brain Res., 11, 111-116.

Besedovsky, H.O., A. del Rey and E. Sorkin (1983a). In: Immunoregulation, Plenum Press, New York, 315-339.

Besedovsky, H.O., A. del Rey and E. Sorkin (1983b). Immunology Today, 4, 342-346.

Besedovsky, H.O., A. del Rey, E. Sorkin, M. da Prada, R. Burri and C. Honesser (1983c). Science, 221, 564-566.

Blalock, J.E., D. Harbour-McMenamin and E.M. Smith (1985). J. Immunol, 135 (suppl.), 858-861.

Blalock, J.E. and E. Smith (1985). Federation Proc., 44, 108-111.

Bloch, B., P. Brazeau, N. Ling, P. Bohlen, F. Esch, W.B. Wehrenberg, R. Benoit, F. Bloom and R. Guillemin (1983). Nature, 306, 607-608.

Brown, W.R.A., A.N. Barclay, C.A. Sunderland and A.F. Williams (1981). Nature, 289, 456-460.Bullock, K., and N.Y. Moore (1981). Am. J. Anat., 162, 157-164.

Cotmore, S.F., S.A. Crowhurst and M.D. Waterfield (1981). Eur. J. Immunol., 11, 597-603.

Crary, B., M. Borysenko, D.C. Sutherland, I. Kutz, J.Z. Borysenko and H. Benson (1983). J. Immunol., 130, 694-697.

Cross, R.S., W.R. Monkesbery, W.M. Brooks and T.L. Roszman (1980). Brain Res., 196, 79-86.

de Tribolet, N., M.F. Hamou, J.P. Mach, S. Carrel and M. Schreyer (1984a). J. Neurol. Neurosurg. Psychiatry, 47, 417-422.

de Tribolet, N., V. piguet, A.C. Diserens, J.P. Mach and S. Carrel (1984b). In: Developmental Neuroscience: Physiological, Pharmacological and Clinical aspects, Elsevier Sc. publ., Amsterdam, 273-279.

Dinarello, C.A. (1984). Rev. Infect. Dis. 6, 51-56.

Dulbecco, R., M. Unser, M. Bologna, H. Battifora, P. Syka and S. Okada (1981). Nature, 292, 772-774.

Engel, W.K., J.L. Trotter, D.E. McFarlin and C.L. McIntosh (1977). Lancet, 1, 1310-1311.

Fabris, N., E. Garaci, J. Hadden and N.A. Mitchison (1983). Immunoregulation, Plenum Press, New York.

Felten, D.L., S.Y. Felten, S.L. Carlson, J.A. Olschowka and S. Livnat (1985). J. Immunol., 135 (suppl.), 755-765.

Fontana, A., F. Kristensen, R. Dubs, D. Gemsa, E. Weber (1982). J. Immunol., 129, 2413-2419.

Fontana, A., K.P.W.J. McAdam, F. Kristensen and F. Weber (1983). Eur. J. Immunol., 13, 685-689.

Fontana, A., W. Fierz and H. Wekerle (1984). Nature, 307, 273-276.

Fontana, A. and W. Fierz (1985). Springer Semin. Immunopathol., 8, 57-70.

Forni, G., M. Bindoni, A. Santoni, N. Belluardo, A.E. Marchese and M. Giovarelli (1983). Nature, 306, 181-184.

Forni, G., M. Bindoni, A. Santoni, M. Giovarelli and A. Mantovani (1984). J. Psychiat. Res., 4, 491-499.

Fuchs, S., S. Schmidt-Hopfeld, G. Tridente and R. Tarrab-Hazdai (1980). Nature, 287, 162-164.

Ghali, W.M., S. Abdel-Rahman, M. Nashib and Z.Y. Mahran (1980). Acta Anat., 108, 115-120.

Ghanta, V.K., R.N. Hiramoto, H.B. Solvason and N.H. Spector (1985). J. Immunol., 135 (suppl.), 848-852.

Goetzl, E.J., T. Chernov, F. Renold and D.G. Payan (1985). J. Immunol., 135 (suppl.), 802-811.

Grossman, Z. (1984) Immunol. Rev., 79, 119-138.

Hall, N.R. and A.L. Goldstein (1983). In; Immunoregulation, Plenum Press, New York, 141-163.

Hall, N.R., J.P. McGillis, B.L. Spangelo and A.L. Goldstein (1985a). J. Immunol., 135 (suppl.), 806-811.

Hall, R.N., J.P. McGillis, B.L. Spangelo, D.L. Healy and A.L. Goldstein (1985b). Springer Semin. Immunopathol., 5, 153-164.

Haynes, B.F. and G.S. Heisenbarth (1983). In: Monoclonal Antibodies: Probes for the Study of Autoimmunity and Immunodeficiency, Academic Press, New York, 48-65.

Hayry, P., E. Willebrand and L.C. Anderson (1980). Scan. J. Immunol., 11, 305-309.

Healy, D.L., G.D. Hodgen, H.M. Schultz, G.P. Chrousos, D.L. Loriaux and R.N. Hall (1983). Science, 222, 1353-1355.

Holboryow, E.J. (1981). Autoimmunity, Saunders, London.

Janeway, C.A., K. Bottomly, J. Babich, P. Conrad, S. Conzen, B. Jones, J. Kaye, M. Katz, L. McVay, D.B. Murphy and J. Tite (1984). Immunology Today, 5, 99-105.

Jerne, N.K. (1974). Ann. Immunol. (Inst. Pasteur), 125C, 373-389.

Johnson, H.M. and B.A. Torres (1985). J. Immunol., 135 (suppl.), 773-775.

Kimelberg, H.K. (1983). Cell. Mol. Neurobiol., 3, 1-8.

Krueger, J., C. Dinarello, L. Wolff, L. Chedis and J. Walter (1984). Am. J. Physiol., 246, R994-998.

Kunkel, H.G. (1983). In: The Biology of Immunologic Diseases, Sinauer, Sunderland, Mass., 247-256.

Leibowitz, S. and R.A.C. Hughes (1983). Immunology of the Nervous System, E. Arnold, London.

Maddox, J. (1984). Nature, 309, 400.

Marx, J.L. (1985) Science, 227, 1190-1192.

Mathews, P.M., C.J. Froehlich, W.L. Sibbitt and A.D. Bankhurst (1983). J. Immunol., 130, 1658-1662.

McGarry, R.C., S.L. Helfond, R.H. Quarles and J.C. Roder (1983). Nature, 306, 376-378.

Moeller, G. (1984). Idiotypic Networks. Immunol. Rev., 79, Munksgaard, Copenhagen.

Moretta, L., C. Mingari and A. Moretta (1982). Sem. Hematol., 19, 273-284.

O'Dorisio, M.S., C.L. Wood and T.M. O'Dorisio (1985). J. Immunol., 135 (suppl.), 792-796.

Payan, D.G. and E.J. Goetzl (1985). J. Immunol., 135 (suppl.), 783-786.

Pert, C.B., M.R. Ruff, R.J. Weber and H. Herkenham (1985). J. Immunol, 135 (suppl.), 820-826.

Pizzighella, S., A.P. Riviera, S. Fuchs, D. Mochly-Rosen and G. Tridente (1982). Protides of the Biological Fluids, Pergamon Press, Oxford, 30, 95-97.

Plotnikoff, N.P. and A.J. Murso (1985). Federation Proc., 44, 91-122.

Pober, J.S., M.A. Gimbrone, R.S. Cotran, C.S. Reiss, S.J. Burakoff, W. Fiers and K.A. Ault (1983). J. Exp. Med., 157, 1339-1353.

Raimond, F., E. Morel and J.F. Bach (1984). J. Neuroimmunol.,6, 31-40.

Renoux, G. (1984). Immunology Today, 5, 218.

Riviera, A.P., S. Pizzighella, E. Nardelli, A. Spiazzi, T. Cestari, F. Paiola and G. Tridente (1985). Protides of the Biological Fluids, Pergamon Press, Oxford, 33 (in press).

Roitt, I., J. Brostoff and D.K. Male (1985). Immunology, Mosby, Saint Louis.

Roszman, T.L., J.C. Jackson, R.J. Cross, M.J. Titus, W.R. Markesbery and W.H. Brooks (1985). J. Immunol., 135 (suppl.), 769-772.

Saris, S.C., S.H. Bigner and D.D. Bigner (1984). J. Neurosurg., 60, 582-589.

Schnegg, J.F., N. de Tribolet, A.C. Diserens, A. Martin-Achard and S. Carrel (1981). Intern. J. Cancer, 28, 265-269.

Schuller-Petrovic, S., W. Gebhart, H. Lassman, H. Rumfold and D. Kroff (1983). Nature, 306, 179-181.

Schwyzer, M. and A. Fontana (1985). J. Immunol., 134, 1003-1009.

Singh, U. (1979). J. Anat., 129, 279-292.

Smith, E.M. and J.E. Blalock (1981). Proc. Nat. Acad. Sci., 30, 78-85.

Smith, E.M., D. Harbour-McMenamin and E.J. Blalock (1985). J. Immunol., 135 (suppl.), 779-782.

Snow, E.C., T.L. Feldbush and J.A. Oaks (1981). J. Immunol., 126, 161-164.

Spector, N.H. (1983). in: Immunoregulation, Plenum Press, New York, 231-258.

Spiess, J., J. Rivier and W. Vale (1983). Nature, 303, 532-535.

Steck, A.J. and N. Murray (1985). Springer Semin. Immunopathol., 8, 29-43.

Stein, M., R.C. Schiavi and M. Camerino (1976). Science, 191, 435-440.

Tridente, G., G.C. Andrighetto, S. Beltrame, F. Gerosa, A. Pezzini, R. Quaini, G. Palestro, E. Leonardi, E. Poggio, G. Maggi and C. Casadio (1978). In: Developments in Clinical Immunology, Academic Press, London, 81-103.

Tridente, G. (1985). Sem. Hematol., 22, 56-67.

Tridente, G., A.P. Riviera, B. Dipasquale, C. Marcon, M. Rocca and M. Gerosa (1985), this volume.

Waksman, B. (1984). Immunology Today, 5, 346-348.

White, F.P., G.R. Dutton and M.D. Norenberg (1981). J. Neurochem.,36, 328-332.

Williams, A.F. (1982). J. theor. Biol., 98, 221-234.

Williams, A.F. and J. Gagnon (1982). Science, 216, 696-703.

Wong, G.H.W., P.F. Bartlett, T. Clark-Lewis, F. Battye and J.W. Schrader (1984). Nature, 310, 688-691.

Wybran, J. (1985). Federation Proc., 44, 92-94.

Antigen Sharing by Glioma Cells and the Epithelial Thymus, as Revealed by the GE$_2$ Monoclonal Antibody

G. Tridente*, A. P. Riviera*, B. Dipasquale*,
C. Marcon*, M. Rocca*, M. Chilosi**
and M. Gerosa***

*Institute of Immunological Sciences, University of Verona,
Verona, Italy
**Department of Pathology, University of Verona, Verona, Italy
***Department of Neurosurgery, University of Verona,
Verona, Italy

KEYWORDS

GE$_2$; monoclonal antibody; thymus; epithelium; glioma.

INTRODUCTION

In recent years evidence has been accumulated regarding a substantial sharing of antigens and receptors by the central nervous system (CNS) and the immune system (IS). Molecules and receptors pertaining to the former have been identified on cells of the latter and vice versa (for general ref. see Tridente, this volume). These findings were initially considered to be apparently irrelevant cross-reactions, possibly important for the pathogenesis of certain autoimmune diseases (Waksman, 1984). Thy-1 molecules, for example, are expressed by rodent thymocytes, human epithelial thymic cells, neuronal cells, fibroblasts, myoblasts and hemopoietic stem cells. Alternatively, such wide distribution has suggested a general role in cell interaction and communication (Williams, 1982).

Coincidental and partial cross-antigenicity could be initially ascribed to these reactions because of the difficulty encountered in isolating and purifying the antigens involved as well as in defining strict identities by polyclonal multi-specific antibodies. High-resolution biochemical purification, amino-acid sequencing and the application of monoclonal antibodies to these studies have revealed striking homologies between Thy-1 antigens, HLA products and immuno-globulins (Barclay and Ward, 1982; Williams and Gagnon, 1982), all of which are now considered members of the immunoglobulin superfamily (Marchalonis et al, 1984). In addition, neuromediators and immune mediators, including specific hormones and receptors, have recently revealed their presence in the CNS and IS, thus leading to the hypothesis of a specific physiological role of these molecules in homeostasis (Goetzl, 1985; Plotnikoff and Murso, 1985).

The occasional observation of Stephan Carrel and associates (de Tribolet et al,

1984) that the GE_2 anti-glioma monoclonal antibody could stain the normal
thymus, among other tissues, prompted us to investigate more carefully the
localization of such specificity within normal and pathologic (from myasthenic
and thymoma-bearing patients) thymuses.

We have found that the GE_2 antibody binds specifically to thymic epithelial
cells which are mainly localized in the cortex (Tridente, 1985). Comparative
analysis with other thymic epithelial cell markers confirms the selectivity of
the binding. Moreover, the presence of this specificity is retained by the adult
myasthenic thymus, albeit with different patterns.

MATERIALS AND METHODS

Fresh frozen sections of normal (chest surgery) or pathologic thymuses were
obtained in the cryostat, dried and fixed with cold chloroform/acetone. Sections
were dipped into phosphate-buffered saline (PBS) and incubated with proper
dilutions of antibody in a moist chamber for 30 min at room temperature,
followed by washing in PBS and a second incubation (30 min) with a peroxidase
conjugated anti-mouse immunoglobulin under the same conditions. Exogenous peroxidase staining was performed with diaminobenzidine or alkaline phosphatase.
Further details regarding the technique and source of antibodies are reported
elsewhere (Chilosi et al, 1985; Nathrath et al, 1985). Some of the sections were
counterstained with conventional hematoxylin.

RESULTS

Using a panel of antisera, reported in Table 1, it is possible to operate a fine
selection of the cellular components of the human thymus. Such a panel is presently employed in this laboratory for studying the histopathology of the
thymus.

The GE_2 pattern is depicted in Figure 1, in which it has been compared in
particular with two other epithelial cell markers, the monoclonal antibody MR3
and the specifically anti-TPA polyclonal antibody.

The specificity of GE_2 for the normal cortical epithelium is clearly shown in
Figure 1a, in which peroxidase-positive cells are encountered at the cortico-
medullary junction. By contrast, the medulla is almost devoid of positive cells.
At higher magnification (Fig. 1b), a delicate network of GE_2-positive cells is
detectable, with a faint borderline positivity for the subcapsular epithelium
and for the outer surface of Hassall's bodies.

In the myasthenic hyperplastic thymus (Fig. 1c), the presence of GE_2 positivity
(here stained with alkaline phosphatase) is confirmed, is more diffuse and
appears to be more pronounced in the medulla as compared to the normal thymus.
However, the medullary positivity (Fig. 1d), here obtained by
peroxidase-hematoxylin double staining, is also to be ascribed to the presence
of dendritic cells of the lymphoid follicles, a typical pathologic lesion of
myasthenic thymuses (Pizzighella et al, 1983).

Finally, Figures 1e and 1f compare positivities obtained with the MR3 and
anti-TPA antibodies respectively, which alternatively show selected positivities

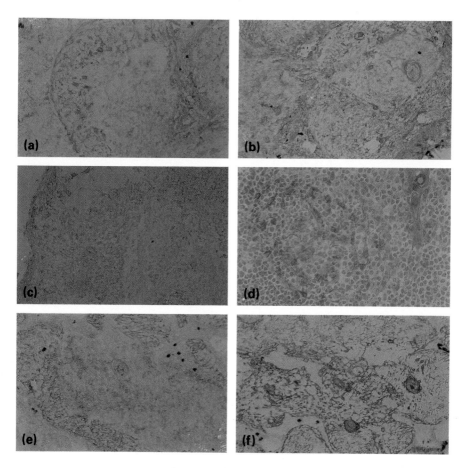

Fig. 1.   Immunohistochemical Pictures
GE$_2$ staining (1a): normal thymus (PAP technique); (1b): same, at higher magnification; (1c): myasthenic hyperplastic thymus (acid phosphatase); (1d): same, using a double staining with peroxidase and hematoxylin. MR3 staining (1e) and TPA staining (1f). (See text for details).

on cortical or medullary (and Hassall's) epithelium. In no case was positivity for thymocytes observed with GE_2.

Table 1. Human Thymus: Immunohistochemical Characterization.

Markers	TdT	CD1 (T6)	CD3 (T3)	TPA	HLA/DR	RFD/4	MR3	KERATIN I	KERATIN II	KERATIN III	DRC	GE_2
Thymocytes												
Subcapsular	+++	–	–	–	–	–	–	–	–	–	–	–
Cortical	++	+++	+	–	–	–	–	–	–	–	–	–
Medullary	–	–	+++	–	–	–	–	–	–	–	–	–
Epithelium												
Subcapsular	–	–	–	+	+/–	++	+/–	++	–	–	–	+
Cortical	–	–	–	–	+++	–	+++	+/–	–	–	–	+++
Medullary	–	–	–	++	+/–	++	+/–	++	–	–	–	–
Hassall's c.	–	–	–	++	–	–	–	–	–	++	–	+
Dendritic cells												
Medullary	–	–	–	–	++	–	–	–	–	–	–	–
Follicular	–	–	–	–	+	–	–	–	–	–	+++	–

+, ++, +++, – = arbitrary positivity scores for each thymus component.

DISCUSSION

These preliminary data clearly show that the presence of GE_2 antigen is selectively located on the cortical thymic epithelium, with a distribution similar to, though stronger than, that of MR3 antibody, particularly at the cortico-medullary junction.

In addition, this positivity is present and accentuated in myasthenic hyperplastic thymuses (non-thymomatous). The positivity on dendritic follicular cells is of great help in individuating follicular structures within the medulla, especially in initial hyperplastic stages where small, isolated follicles are difficult to detect by conventional histopathology. It should be noted that positivity for dendritic cells has already been noted in lymph nodes (de Tribolet et al, 1984). Employing the panel of antisera reported in Table 1, we are extending these studies to thymoma (with or without myasthenia) where thymic epithelial anomalies have already been documented (Chilosi et al, 1985). The relation of GE_2 antigens to other common neuro-immune antigens such as Thy-1 remains to be ascertained.

ACKNOWLEDGEMENTS AND NOTES

This work was supported in part by the Italian National Research Council under the Oncology Research Project, by the Ministry of Education and by ARBI, Verona. These data were presented by the author at the Meeting as part of his review of interactions between the central nervous and immune systems.

REFERENCES

Barclay, A.N. and H.A. Ward (1982). Eur. J. Biochem., 129, 447-458.
Chilosi, M., A. Iannucci, L. Fiore-Donati, G. Tridente, M. Pampanini, G. Pizzolo, M. Ritter, M. Bofill and G. Janossy (1985). J. Neuroimmunol., in press.
de Tribolet, N., V. Piguet, A.C. Diserens, J.P. Mach and S. Carrel (1984). In: Developmental Neuroscience: Physiological, Pharmacological and Clinical Aspects, Elsevier Sci. Publ., Amsterdam, 273-279.
Goetzl, E.J. (1985). J. Immunol., 135 (suppl.).
Marchalonis, J.J., G.R. Vasta, G.W. Warr and W.C. Barker (1984). Immunology Today, 5, 133-142.
Nathrath, W.B.J., P. Heidenkummer, V. Bjoerklund and B. Bjoerklund (1985). J. Histochem. Biochem., 33, 99-109.
Pizzighella, S., A.P. Riviera and G. Tridente (1983). J. Neuroimmunol., 4, 117-127.
Plotnikoff, N.P. and A.J. Murso (1985). Federation Proc., 44, 91-122.
Tridente, G. (1985), this volume.
Tridente, G. (1985). Sem. Hematol., 22, 56-67.
Waksman, B. (1985). Immunology Today, 5, 346-348.
Williams, A.F. (1982). J. theor. Biol., 98, 221-234.
Williams, A.F. and J. Gagnon (1982). Science,216, 696-703.

In Vitro Models as Guides to Clinical Chemotherapy

J. S. Kovach

Department of Oncology, Mayo Clinic, Rochester,
Minnesota, USA

ABSTRACT

The reasons underlying the relative ineffectiveness of chemotherapy of the most
common solid tumors are not known. The relationship, if any, of "intrinsic"
resistance to drugs such as shown by colon cancer to "acquired" resistance to
drugs in which initial success is followed by progression in the face of the
same therapy as typified by carcinomas of the head and neck is not known. In
the absence of an understanding of the mechanisms underlying "clinical drug
resistance" an understanding of the relationships between cytotoxicity of drugs
in vitro to success or lack of success with the same drugs in vivo may not be
possible. Indeed, without an understanding of the effects of a given drug regimen at the cellular level in vivo, potentially useful drugs and possibly important biological prinicples may be overlooked. Certainly, with rare exceptions,
the mechanisms responsible for resistance of tumors at the clinical level are
not known to be related to the same mechanims of resistance which have been
described in innumerable in vitro systems.

The hope that measurement of one parameter or another of cell growth in vitro in
the presence and absence of a given drug or group of drugs would provide information relevant to the selection of therapy for an individual patient has not
been realized. On the other hand, although multiple drugs and combinations of
drugs have been demonstrated to have marked activity against a variety of tumor
cells in vitro, this information has not led to the development of improved
therapeutic regimens with few exceptions. Many theories and model systems have
been advanced to explain the failure at the clinical level of drug regimens
active in vitro and to some extent in vivo in animal models. Thus, drug
resistance has been ascribed to differences in cell kinetics and to genetically
determined differences such as drug transport, activation, efflux, and/or in
capabilities of repair. Although these mechanisms may in fact limit the effectiveness in vivo of many drug regimens active at the clinical level is simply a matter of drug delivery to
the intended target. Although assessment of drug concentration and drug action
at the cellular level is difficult clinically, failure to exclude drug delivery
as a primary cause of therapeutic failure will perpetuate the belief that differences in the effectiveness of drugs against cell lines in vitro and against
the same types of cells growing in vivo are caused by fundamental differences in
the biochemical nature of the targets rather than by differences in delivery of

drug to the targets. Recent advances in biochemical, immunochemical, and histologic techniques should make it possible to determine to what extent delivery of
amounts of drug insufficient to produce cytotoxic effects underlies "clinical
drug resistance."

INTRODUCTION

In 1977, Hamburger and Salmon reported the potential value of a "human tumor
stem cell assay" (HTSCA) for measuring the chemosensitivity of primary human
tumors. Although the number of laboratories carrying out the assay has proli-
ferated markedly, lack of proliferation of primary tumor cells in vitro, among
other factors, continues to limit prospective clinical evaluation of the method
as a useful clinical tool. This review provides one point of view concerning
the present status of the HTSCA and discusses additional approaches to the goal
of a better understanding of the chemosensitivity of primary human tumors.

In the soft agar assay, attempts at measurement of drug sensitivity are based on
inhibition of one or another parameter of the integrity or function of cells
derived from mechanically or enzymatically disrupted tumors (Mattern and Volm,
1982; Salmon, 1984; Twentyman, 1985). The concept underlying the use of cells
from primary human tumors to study drug sensitivity in vitro in a manner analogous to methods used for the determination of drug sensitivity of infectious
agents is highly appealing. The expectation is that in vitro, patterns of sensitivity of cells from primary tumors reflect the in vivo sensitivities of those
tumors and will provide a guide to selection of active chemotherapeutic regimens
or, at least, a guide for exclusion of ineffective drugs. After the initial in
vitro studies of cells from primary human tumors were carried out, several
groups reported retrospective correlations between in vitro sensitivity and in
vivo sensitivity (Salmon et al, 1978; Alberts et al, 1980; Von Hoff, 1981).
These early claims encouraged numerous laboratories to develop the assay within
their own institutions.

Until recently, most studies did not address in any detail the important issue
of how to simulate in vitro the complex metabolic and structural features which
tumors possess in vivo. It was assumed that the appearance of masses of cellular material, initially called clones, in soft agar upon incubation of cells
disrupted from primary tumors represented proliferation of tumor stem cells. It
was believed that the presence of fewer larger "colonies" in the presence of one
or another drug reflected intrinsic sensitivity of the primary tumor to the
antiproliferative activity of the drug producing the reduction in colony formation. Over several years, it has become apparent that, for the most part,
clusters of colonies of cells found in the soft agar assay after the introduction of material from disrupted primary tumors arise from clumps of cells rather
than from individual cells and, therefore, are not clonal in origin (Agrez et
al, 1982; Selby et al, 1983). Others, particularly Schlag and Schreml, 1982,
have emphasized that there are marked differences in cloning efficiencies and
chemosensitivities of primary human tumors and metastases from those tumors
using standard soft agar assays. They point out that one cannot be certain if
these differences are methodological or biological in origin.

ASSAYS BASED ON COLONY FORMATION

It is only in the past few years that it has been appreciated that the relationship of chemosensitivity data obtained in the soft agar assay of cells
derived from primary human tumors to the tumor in vivo is very difficult to
establish primarily because there is no possibility to repeat studies to confirm
initial results. Given this situation, every effort must be made to document
and establish the reliability of the assay by employing the most rigorous
controls in each experiment. Several requirements are obvious but merit
discussion because they are frequently omitted or given only cursory treatment

in reports of results of in vitro chemosensitivity studies. It is necessary to have an accurate determination of the number of clusters of cells initially placed in the assay and of the extent of variability in that number. That is, variability in control plates and in experimental plates must be documented so that differences occurring in the presence of drug can be placed in the context of the degree of experimental error. Furthermore, for each tumor studied, the endpoints, whether incorporation of radiolabel or number of colonies, should be documented to fall within the linear range of the assay. It is difficult if not impossible to make comparisons between experimental and control values if this is not the case.

The importance of experimentally determining the linear range of the colony forming assay of primary human tumor cells in each experimental situation has been largely ignored in the past. Recently, Eliason et al (1985) found that the cloning efficiency of 51 primary tumor samples was independent of cell number for only 53% of samples. The other samples varied equally between those in which cloning efficiency increased and those in which cloning efficiency decreased with increasing cell input. They concluded that dependence of cloning efficiency upon number of cells plated should be examined in each experiment particularly in studies in which effects of drugs are to be measured.

Of equal importance to linearity of the assay, is the need for positive controls in each assay. It must be possible to determine precisely the "background" which represents total inhibition of whatever parameter of cell function or integrity is being used to assess drug sensitivity. One approach adopted by many investigators has been to eliminate from consideration experiments in which variability in control plates and in the absolute number of "objects" present in control plates exceeds certain predetermined "acceptable" values. It is not at all clear that exclusion of experiments in which variability is marked does not introduce an important selection bias. Virtually no studies in the literature discuss the basis for marked variability in replicate plates in some experiments other than to suggest that this is always the result of poor disaggregation of the primary tumor.

Finally, it must be shown that drug effects in the assay are dose-dependent. This point has been made by many investigators, perhaps most forcefully by Selby et al (1983).

The greatest effort to date to validate and standardize a soft agar assay of primary tumor cell sensitivity was reported by Shoemaker et al (1985). In a series of extensive studies and refinements of assay technique, they present data which indicate that nontoxic compounds have little or no activity as measured by inhibition of the formation of colonies of a variety of primary tumors in vitro and that drugs known to be cytotoxic to mammalian cells do inhibit formation of colonies by cells from some primary human tumor cells in vitro. These findings support the belief that measurement of numbers of cell clusters in soft agar reflects sensitivity of the clusters to a specific cytotoxic environment. However, the data also raise concerns about variability within the test system. A particular concern is that in the initial blinded trial of multiple drugs, the positive control (sodium azide at 600 μg/ml) was "cytotoxic" in only 28% of the studies. In a subsequent blinded study, mercuric chloride (100 μg/ml) was substituted for sodium azide. This compound, which is believed to be highly cytotoxic, was positive in only 34 of 65 separate assays (52%). The reasons why mercuric chloride and sodium azide are not uniformly effective in reducing colony formation are not known and apparently have not been studied.

One must consider the possibility that random variability in assay methodology rather than unusual biology is the basis for these results. This possiblity is supported by large variations in the activity of individual drugs in 2 blinded experiments reported by Shoemaker et al (1985). In the initial study, cisplatin produced responses in 17 of 70 tumors (24%). In a second blinded trial, the response rate for cisplatin was 30 of 56 (54%). The response rates for melphalan varied between the 2 studies from 10% to 21%. These kinds of differences are not surprising given the variability inherent in the assay. However, differences of 100% or more in the frequency of activity of a given compound may be large enough to make determination of the significance of activity against any one tumor difficult and complicates significantly interpretation of results for screening purposes.

ASSAYS BASED ON INHIBITION OF SYNTHESIS OF MACROMOLECULES

Variability in disruption of tumor cells, inability to obtain clonal growth, and difficulties in detecting truly proliferative colonies in semisolid medium against a background of hundreds of thousands of single cells and clusters of cells, have led a number of investigators to study methods other than enumeration of the formation of clusters of cells as a means of assessing cytotoxic effects of drugs. Most popular at the moment, is measurement of inhibition of incorporation of radiolabeled substrates into protein or nucleic acids (Tanigawa et al, 1982; Sondak et al, 1984; Jones et al, 1985). Inhibition of thymidine incorporation into acid-precipitable material has been studied most extensively. The assumption underlying these assays is that inhibition of incorporation of amino acids and/or nucleic acid analogs in cells from disaggregated tumors by drugs reflects the sensitivity to those drugs of tumors in vivo.

Most assays using incorporation of a radiolabeled substrate are carried out over a relatively short period of time during which most tumor cells undergo less than one cell division. During this period, many cells including non-stem cells of the tumor cell population and any other viable cells present such as fibroblasts may contribute to the final result expressed as amount of radioactivity per experimental unit. To expect that this type of measurement will reflect the character of the target cell population in vivo seems optimistic. Despite these concerns, the value of such a method for ascertaining in vivo tumor drug resistance is so appealing that this approach has merited considerable attention.

Mattern and Volm (1982) have recently reviewed "in vitro/in vivo" correlations with 3 types of assays: measurement of cellular damage in monolayer and organ cultures, measurement of inhibition of incorporation of radiolabeled precursors predominantly uridine and thymidine, and inhibition of colony formation. In general, there appears to be an in vitro/in vivo correlation of sensitivity ranging from 45% to 78% and of resistance of approximately 95% in all 3 assay systems. These numbers raise hopes that in vitro assessments of "drug sensitivity" will have some impact upon the therapeutics of cancer. As discussed earlier, however, virtually none of the reported assays included effective positive controls and did not address the linearity of the assay for each tumor as would appear to be necessary from the data of Eliason et al (1985). Similarly, most reports do not discuss variability among replicates of experimental plates compared to the variability among replicates of control plates so as to make it possible to assess the significance of the magnitude of differences between experimental points and control points. Such requirements may seem too demanding given the limitations of the assay in terms of availability of tumor material. However, because in virtually none of these studies are experiments repeatable, it is necessary to insist on the most rigorous of controls to establish to the extent possible the reliability of measurements.

One of the largest studies utilizing incorporation of thymidine as the measure of drug effect was recently reported by Sondak et al (1984). They added 5 μCi of tritiated thymidine (~ 5,000,000 cpm at 50% efficiency counting) to each plate to label the thymidine pool. They considered an assay evaluable if "untreated control" plates had 300 cpm more than "background" plates to which 600 µg/ml of sodium azide had been added. It should be recalled that sodium azide at this concentration had been rejected as an effective positive control by the cooperative group study reported by Shoemaker et al (1985) in which colony counting was the endpoint because sodium azide was positive in only 28% of tumors. In the study of Sondak et al (1984), 142/219 tumors gave "sensitivity" data; 33 of 142 provided in vitro/in vivo correlations. Thirteen of the 33 tumors were considered sensitive in vitro and 20 of the 33 tumors were considered resistant in vitro. None of the 20 tumors with in vitro resistance responded to therapy. It should be noted that 15 of these 20 patients were treated with single agent chemotherapy and 5 patients were treated with 3- or 4-drug-combination therapy. Of the 13 patients whose tumors were determined to be sensitive in vitro, 5 patients (39%) were judged to have partial regressions to 3- or 4-drug-combinations and one patient had stabilization of disease to a 4-drug-regimen. Seven of the 13 patients whose tumors were sensitive in vitro failed to respond to treatment. Five of these failed to respond to treatment with a single agent and 2 failed to respond to treatment with a 3- or 4-drug-combination regimen. Thus, of attempts to study 219 solid tumor specimens using thymidine incorporation as a measure of drug sensitivity, 13 patients met the criteria established for in vitro sensitivity, (9 of these were "sensitive" to 3- or 4-drug combinations). Of these 13, less than half were judged to have a partial objective response.

These results are similar to those of the largest prospective study (Von Hoff et al, 1983) in which inhibition of colony formation rather than inhibition of thymidine incorporation was used to determine chemosensitivity. In this study, assays were considered to be adequate for drug sensitivity testing if there were an average of 20 colonies per 500,000 nucleated cells plated. Single agent therapy was selected for patients on the basis of the drug producing the greatest degree of inhibition of colony formation regardless of the extent of that inhibition. Of 246 "single-agent studies" in which drug was administered on the basis of in vitro results of the cloning assay, the overall response rate was 25%. In 358 single agent-trials in which the drug choice was made by the responsible physician, the overall response rate was 15% and in a group of patients who either refused or who had a clinical reason preventing administration of the drug indicated by the assay, the response rate was 11%. The study was not randomized and, as the authors point out, no meaningful comparisons of these low response rates can be made. However, the data from this trial and from that of Sondak et al (1984) demonstrate the difficulties in assessing the potential clinical value of in vitro assays of drug sensitivity as currently practiced.

Despite an apparent striking correlation of in vitro drug resistance to in vivo resistance there is little evidence supporting the contention that the in vitro assay is measuring a parameter relevant to clinical responsiveness. Because most solid tumors are relatively unresponsive to any chemotherapy, particularly single agent chemotherapy, it is not surprising that using arbitrary criteria for classifying in vitro responses as sensitive or resistant, high degrees of correlation of in vitro results with therapeutic failure, may be found. Correlations of approximately 50% with respect to clinical response of tumors judged to be sensitive in vitro have in several instances relied upon clinical responses to combinations of drugs, although no one has addressed the issue of how to mimic in vitro the effects of multiple drugs in vivo. At the present time, it appears that in vitro assays of the drug sensitivity of primary human tumor cells do not have a role in patient management that can be justified on the basis of current data (Salmon et al, 1984; Bradley et al, 1984; Schlag and Flentje, 1984). Several groups have expressed interest in using in vitro assays of primary human tumor cells as a broad screen looking for antitumor activity of new compounds which are not detected by conventional screens. Present data suggests that before this approach can be tested in a meaningful way, there must be greater understanding of the relationship between in vitro proliferation of primary human tumor cells and those characteristics of the tumor which determine responsiveness to chemotherapy in vivo.

ASSAYS USING CELL LINES

An attractive alternative to characterizing and studying mechanisms of tumor resistance is the development of cell lines from primary human tumors before and after development of in vivo clinical resistance. Brain tumors appear to be particularly well suited to this approach since cells from many of brain cancers can be cultured for varying periods of time providing an opportunity investigate in a controlled manner dose-response relationships. The complexities of studying "stem cell sensitivity" of malignant brain tumors in culture have been thoroughly discussed by Rosenblum and Gerosa (1984). Recent advances in defining culture conditions required to propagate primary human tumor cells with high efficiency in vitro raise the possibility that many cell tupes derived from cancers other than brain tumors may be maintained for periods of time in a pro- liferative state in culture sufficiently long to allow characterization of sen- sitivity to multiple drugs and to explore the mechanisms underlying resistance.

Outstanding among such efforts are those of Minna and his colleagues (Gazdar et al, 1980; Carney et al, 1981; Carney et al, 1983) in defining culture conditions required for the proliferation of small cell carcinomas of the lung and more recently other types of carcinoma. Although comprehensive analyses of the chemotherapy sensitivity profiles of most of these lines have not yet been published, there are indications that some morphologic and drug sensitivity parameters are different between cell lines derived from clinically resistant tumors and cell lines derived from clinically sensitive tumors. It is to be hoped that those characteristics of primary solid tumors which are determinants of drug sensitivity will be maintained in cell lines derived from the tumor. However, analysis of the effects of a single drug let alone combinations of drugs upon a heterogeneous cell population obtained after disruption of highly organized cellular material whose structure and perhaps even synthesis of specialized molecules such as growth factors might be crucial for integrity and proliferation, seems to pose a level of complexity not approachable by measure- ment of cell growth in culture. The difficulties encountered with in vitro systems as models predictive for the clinic have led us to reassess the value of in vivo animal models for discovery of new drugs and for designing clinically effective regimens.

ANIMAL MODELS FOR DEVELOPING CLINICAL CHEMOTHERAPY REGIMENS

Because many regimens active in in vivo model systems have failed to produce dramatic responses clinically, there is a tendency to believe that the animal models do not reflect the biological factors which are important in determining clinical response. Usually, a chemotherapeutic regimen is declared inactive or more often, a tumor is said to be "drug-resistant" clinically even though the reasons for failure of the regimen clinically are not known. That is, the biologic and pharmacologic conditions achieved in the model systems in which a chemotherapeutic regimen produces "activity" are not known to have been repro- duced in the tumor target in man. In the absence of knowledge of, at least, the intracellular concentrations of the active forms of the drugs in the model systems and in the intended targets in man, assessment of relevance of any model to the clinic cannot be made with certainty.

Murine leukemia is regarded by many investigators as a useful model for the development of regimens effective against human leukemia because a number of drugs active against mouse leukemia in vivo have activity against human leukemia (Skipper, 1978). The opposite situation is true for solid tumors. Many drugs tested against and showing activity against solid tumor models in the mouse do not have "comparable" degrees of activity against solid tumors in man. The failure of these drugs to produce clinical responses in man does not necessarily mean that murine solid tumor models are not useful models for man. In general, solid tumor models in the mouse have been selected as test systems because they are reproducibly responsive in a dose dependent manner to at least some anticancer drugs. These models almost invariably involve transplantation of cell suspensions or clusters of cells followed by drug treatment shortly after transplantation. Many drugs demonstrate activity against many different types of solid tumors in the mouse under such experimental conditions. By and large endpoints such as delay in tumor growth are used rather than tumor regression and long-term survivorship. Drugs showing activity in such models are taken to the clinic, not to be tested against the initial growth phases of rapidly proliferating transplanted cancer, but in most cases to be evaluated for activity against advanced disease. When the model tumors in mice are allowed to proceed to a state comparable to advanced tumors in man, many drugs active against these tumors at early stages of development do not produce dramatic therapeutic effects if therapeutic effects.

Because we are constrained clinically to assess new drug regimens predominantly against advanced cancers, it seems reasonable to test the possibility that the appropriate model systems for advanced disease in man are advanced solid tumors in animals. The fact that such tumors in animals are not responsive to even our "best" drugs argues for the potential relevance of advanced disease in the mouse as an appropriate model. Tumors in the mouse which are responsive to a given drug regimen at an early stage of proliferation and which fail to respond to the same regimen when therapy is initiated at an advanced stage of tumor progression may be excellent models for the human situation. At least such tumors allow the possibility of examining mechanisms responsible for resistance as a function of stage of tumor progression. It is not sufficient to assume that all things are equal with respect to drug therapy particularly drug delivery to tumor cell populations at early stages and at advanced stages of tumor progression except for the total mass of tumor.

DRUG DELIVERY AND "CLINICAL" DRUG RESISTANCE

It is beyond the scope of this presentation to consider the multiple mechanisms which may be responsible for the failure of many advanced solid tumors to respond to drugs. Certainly the concepts of intrinisic and/or acquired drug resistance at the genetic level (Goldie and Coldman, 1979; Dembo, 1984) and cell kinetic parameters particularly the existance of large numbers of cells in advanced tumors in a "dormant" state (Carter, 1984) have occupied the attention of many investigators. While these factors have been demonstrated to play a role in determining drug sensitivity in a variety of model systems, less complicated explanations such as failure of drug delivery to large numbers of cells in advanced solid tumors as a primary cause of clinical drug resistance have not been excluded.

There is considerable evidence from in vitro models using spheroids of tumor cells (Sutherland and Durand, 1984), that clusters of tumors with diameters as little as 0.5 mm may pose substantial barriers to distribution of a variety of drugs throughout the tumor mass (Nederman and Twentyman, 1984). Should drug distribution throughout solid tumors in man be a major cause of drug resistance, development of new therapeutic modalities which modify the intercellular matrix and/or cell surface may prove to be essential if we are to develop drug regimens effective against these tumors. These considerations are speculative. However, it seems we should address the issue as to what extent drug delivery to cells growing as monolayers differs from drug delivery to cells growing in 3-dimensional structures as is the case for most solid tumors in vivo. Conversely, we should study those solid tumors in man such as lymphomas and germ cell carcinomas which can be cured by chemotherapy alone even in an advanced

state. We should determine if these tumors present less effective barriers to
drug distribution throughout tumor masses that other solid tumors which cannot
be cured with aggressive chemotherapy. Certainly, in addition to physical
barriers, it is clear that when cells grow in intimate contact with each other,
there are morphologic and presumably biochemical alterations which although not
well defined, are associated with resistance to drugs and to ionizing radiation
(Dertinger et al, 1983; Guichard et al, 1983; Rasey, J.S., 1983; Nederman,
1984). The fact that cells growing as spheroids rather than as monolayers show
increased resistance to ionizing radiation where distribution of therapeutic
modality is not a factor, points out that "cell-cell contact" cannot be ignored
when assessing the effectiveness or lack of effectiveness of a given therapeutic
modality.

With recent advances in analytical methodologies, it is now possible to measure
drug concentrations in small samples of tissue and even in single cells. These
techniques for analysis combined with procedures such as computerized
tomographic directed thin needle biopsy for obtaining tissue samples will permit
the characterization of drug distribution and metabolism in tumors in vivo in
man. This information will make it possible to compare cellular pharmacologic
findings in models to the clinical situation. These comparisons will facilitate
rational development and exploitation of models predictive for the clinic in the
near future.

REFERENCES

Agrez, M.V., J.S. Kovach and M.M. Lieber (1982). Br. J. Cancer, 46, 880-887.
Bradley, E.C., B.F. Issell and R. Hellman (1984). Invest. New Drugs, 2, 59-70.
Carney, D.N., L. Broder, M. Edelstein, A.F. Gazdar, M. Hansen, K. Havemann, M.
    Matthews, G.D. Sorenson and L. Videlov (1983). Cancer Treat. Rep., 67, 27-35.
Carney, E.N., P.A. Bunn Jr., A.F. Gazdar, J.A. Pagan and J.D. Minna (1981).
    Proc. Natl. Acad. Sci., 78, 3185-3189.
Carter, S.K. (1984). Cancer Treat. Rev., 11 (Supplement A), 3-7.
Dembo, A.J. (1984). J. Clin. Oncol., 2, 1311-1316.
Dertinger, H., M. Guichard and E.P. Malaise (1983). Radiat. Environ. Biophys.,
    22, 209-214.
Durand, R.E. and R.M. Sutherland (1984). Spheroids in Cancer Research, Methods
    and Perspectives, Springer-Verlag, Heidelberg, pp. 103-115.
Eliason, J.F., M.S. Aapro, D. Decrey and M. Brink-Petersen (1985). Br. J.
    Cancer, 52, 311-318.
Gazdar, A.F., D.N. Carney, E.K. Russell, H.L. Sims, S.B. Baylin, P.A. Bunn, J.G.
    Guccion and J.D. Minna (1980). Cancer Res., 40, 3502-3507.
Guichard, M., H. Dertinger and E.P. Malaise (1983). Radiat. Res., 95, 602-609.
Jones, C.A., T. Tsukamoto, P.C. O'Brien, C.B. Uhl, M.C. Alley and M.M. Lieber
    (1985). Br. J. Cancer, 52, 303-310.
Mattern, J. and M. Volm (1982). Cancer Treat. Rev., 9, 267-298.
Nederman, T. and P. Twentyman (1984). Spheroids in Cancer Research, Methods
    and Perspectives, Springer-Verlag, Heidelberg, pp. 84-102.
Rasey, J.S. (1983). Proc. Inter. Congr. Radiat. Res., Martinus Nijhoff
    Publishers, pp. 303-310.
Rosenblum, M.L. and M.A. Gerosa (1984). Prog. Exp. Tumor Res., 28, 1-17.
Salmon, S.E. (1984). Cancer Treat. Rep., 68, 117-125.
Salmon, S.E., F.L. Meyskens and D.S. Alberts (1984). Br. J. Cancer, 50,
    725-726.
Schlag, P. and D. Flentje (1984). Cancer Treat. Rev., 11 (Supplement A),
    131-137.
Schlag, P. and W. Schreml (1982). Cancer Res., 42, 4086-4089.
Selby, P., R.N. Buick and I. Tannock (1983). N. Engl. J. Med., 308, 129-134.
Shoemaker, R.H., M.K. Wolpert-DeFilippes, D.H. Kern, M.M. Lieber, R.W. Makuch,
    N.R. Melnick, W.T. Miller, S.E. Salmon, R.M. Simon, J.M. Venditti and D.D. Von
    Hoff (1985). Cancer Res., 45, 2145-2153.

Skipper, H.E. (1978). Cancer Chemotherapy, Volume 1: Reasons for Success and Failure in Treatment of Murine Leukemias With the Drugs Now Employed in Treating Human Leukemias, American Society of Clinical Oncology, Inc., pp. 1-166.

Sondak, V.K., C.A. Bertelsen, N. Tanigawa, S.U. Hildebrand-Zanki, D.L. Morton, E.L. Korn and D.H. Kern (1984). Cancer Res., 44, 1725-1728.

Sutherland, R.M. and R.E. Durand (1984). Spheroids in Cancer Research, Methods and Perspectives, Springer-Verlag, Heidelberg, pp. 24-49.

Tanigawa, N., D.H. Kern, Y. Hikasa and D.L. Morton (1982). Cancer Res., 42, 2159-2164.

Thomas, D.G.T., J.L. Darling, E.A. Paul, T.J. Mott, J.N. Godlee, J.S. Tobias, L.G. Capra, C.D. Collins, C. Mooney, T. Bozek, G.P. Finn, S.O. Arigbabu, D.E. Bullard, N. Shannon and R.I. Freshney (1985). Br. J. Cancer, 51, 525-532.

Twentyman, P.R. (1985). Br. J. Cancer, 51, 295-299.

Wilson, A.P., C.H.J. Ford, C.E. Newman and A. Howell (1984). Br. J. Cancer, 49, 57-63.

In Vitro Short-term Nonclonogenic Assays: an Approach for the Study of the Interactions Between Drugs and Human Tumors

O. Sanfilippo, R. Silvestrini, M. G. Daidone
and N. Zaffaroni

Oncologia Sperimentale C, Istituto Nazionale per lo Studio e la
Cura dei Tumori, Via Venezian 1, 20133 Milan, Italy

ABSTRACT

In the last 20 years different in vitro short-term systems have been proposed
for the preclinical study of drug activity on human tumors. The actual limits
and potentials of the application of these systems to individual patients'
treatment are under investigation, as are new fields of application to some
basic studies on mechanisms of drug-human tumor interaction. As a guideline for
the discussion of fields of application and possible problems related to in
vitro testing on fresh human tumors, the methodologic approach of a short-term
assay used in our laboratory on different human tumor types since 1974 is herein
summarized. Analysis of clinical predictivity based on retrospective and
preliminary prospective clinical trials are reported. Moreover, basic studies
carried out with the assay on interlesion heterogeneity in drug sensitivity and
on patterns of cross-resistance among antitumor drugs are described.

KEY WORDS

Antitumor drugs, in vitro chemosensitivity, human tumors, short-term assays,
clinical correlations, tumor heterogeneity, cross-resistance

INTRODUCTION

In the last 10 years much effort has been made to improve in vitro chemosensitivity tests on human tumors. In addition to the well-known clonogenic assays
proposed by Hamburger and Salmon (1977) and Courtenay, et al (1978), different
approaches have been proposed; they had the main aims of being simple and
successful in a large number of tumors. The latter characteristic appears
essential for the application of the assays to preclinical screening for individual patients. In this paper some general aspects of the nonclonogenic assays
are discussed. Moreover, our experience with a nucleic acid precursor incorporation (NPI) assay we have used since 1974 is reported as a guideline for the
discussion of potentialities for different fields of application and of the
still unsolved problems of in vitro short-term testing.

GENERAL ASPECTS OF SHORT-TERM ASSAYS

Among the nonclonogenic assays, two large subgroups can be considered: the
first one includes the intermediate-term assays in which drug effects are

evaluated after in vitro culture intervals (8) long enough to allow evaluation of the cytocidal effect of the drugs. Most of the more reliable, recently proposed assays require tumor cell suspensions, whereas different biologic markers of drug activity such as changes in cell morphology (Wheeler, et al, 1974), cell viability (Durkin, et al, 1979; Weisenthal, et al, 1983) or uptake of labeled precursors involved in key metabolic processes for cell replication (Dendy, et al, 1981; Sondak, et al, 1985; Thomas, et al, 1985) are used as endpoints of drug activity. Most of these assays have given interesting results in terms of predictivity of in vitro sensitivity on clinical objective response (Wheeler et al, 1974; Bosanquet, et al, 1983; Morasca, et al, 1983; Sondak, et al, 1985) or long-term response to treatment, such as disease-free interval or overall survival (Dendy, 1981; Thomas, et al, 1985). However, possible pitfalls of these assays are linked to selection of subpopulations as well as to blockade in cell cycle progression during the in vitro culture of the freshly prepared cell suspensions.

To the second subgroup belong the short-term assays. Owing to the short times of in vitro culture, these assays do not directly evaluate cytocidal effects but only the drug interference on cell pathways involved in tumor cell replication, such as incorporation of labeled precursors into DNA and RNA (Volm, et al, 1979; Maddox, et al, 1984; Preisler, et al, 1984; Sanfilippo, et al, 1984). Moreover, the short incubation time does not make it possible to reveal long-term mechanism of repair and makes the evaluation of the the effect of phase-specific drugs critical. In any case, these assays are relatively simple and not time-consuming, so that they are suitable for prediction of individual tumor chemosensitivity. Moreover, the adaptability of the test to solid samples and the shortness of in vitro culture greatly reduce the possibility of subpopulation selection and of biologic modifications. Notwithstanding the possible pitfalls, many of these assays proved to be predictive of patient clinical response in retrospective-correlative studies (Daidone, et al, 1981; KSST, 1981; Sanfilippo, et al, 1981; Possinger, et al, 1983; Preisler, et al, 1984; Schwarzmeier, et al, 1984; Silvestrini, et al, 1984).

METHODOLOGY OF THE NPI ASSAY

The technical details of assay, which is based on the evaluation of nucleic acid precursor incorporation into DNA and RNA, have been described (Sanfilippo, et al, 1984) and its essential steps are discussed here in detail. Cell suspensions from effusions or systemic diseases and fragments from solid tumors are used as assay material to avoid possible selection of tumor cell subpopulations during the disaggregation procedures. For each tumor, some random fragments or a sample of the cell suspension is submitted to histologic verification of the correct tumor sampling and to autoradiographic analysis of the incorporation of ^{3}H-thymidine into tumor and nontumor cells. In vitro treatment consists of a 3-h incubation in the presence of drugs at concentrations calculated from the clinical single dose by means of the formula of Tisman (Tisman, et al, 1973): such defined concentrations are generally close to the plasma peak level concentrations. DNA and RNA precursors (^{3}H-thymidine and ^{3}H-uridine) are added to the culture media for 1 h (from the 2nd to the 3rd hour). Nucleic acids are extracted, from pulverized tissue or from cellular pellets, by precipitation in cold (0°C) trichloroacetic acid and separated by alkaline hydrolysis. Radioactivity incorporation is expressed as total dpm for cell suspensions or as incorporation in the nucleic acids relative to the overall cellular uptake for fragments.

Definition of in vitro sensitivity is one of the more crucial points of the in vitro assays. In fact, drug activity may vary from no effect to very high inhibition of the parameter at study, and criteria for the definition of the cutoff point for sensitivity are required for each drug and each tumor type. After preliminary attempts to use retrospective criteria (Daidone, et al, 1981; Sanfilippo, et al, 1981), we adopted prospective criteria (Daidone, et al, 1982;

Silvestrini, et al, 1983) in which both the intratumor heterogeneity, evaluated as variation in incorporation in triplicate control samples, and the intertumor variability in effects of each drug in different tumors with similar histology were taken into account. Feasibility of the NPI assay previously reported (Sanfilippo, et al, 1984) was confirmed on more than 4000 tumors of different histologies, including non-Hodgkin lymphomas (NHL), malignant melanomas (MM), breast cancers (BC), germ cell testicular tumors (GCTT), epithelial ovarian cancers (EOC) and colorectal cancers (CRC) received by our laboratory from 1974 to 1985. The feasibility of the assay ranged from 60% in NHL to a maximum of 92% for CRC, with the exception of operable BC, in which the small size of the tumor and the priority of other biologic determinations limited the feasibility to 15% of the cases.

FIELDS OF APPLICATION

Potentialities of the assay for its use in basic and applied studies of drug-tumor interactions were verified in the last 5 years. The more immediate use of the in vitro assays is to gain preclinical information on drug sensitivities of subgroups as well as of indvidual tumors. With this aim the potential of the assay in predicting clinical sensitivity was investigated in large series of tumors with different morphologic, biologic and pathologic characteristics (Silvestrini, et al, 1984, 1985) and in tumors in which in vitro sensitivity was individually compared to patient response. More recently, the in vitro assay was used to investigate some basic aspects of drug activity such as the inter-lesion heterogeneity in drug sensitivity and the relative activities of similar and unrelated drugs.

EVALUATION OF CLINICAL PREDICTIVITY

The ability of the assay to predict tumor type sensitivity was investigated through different analyses: the ability of the assay to reproduce the peculiar sensitivities of different tumor types to the drugs more conventionally used in clinical trials was first studied. In vitro response rates of tumors with different degrees of clinical chemosensitivity are reported in Table 1. In vitro sensitivity of a clinically chemosensitive tumor, such as NHL, was higher than that observed for a classical clinically resistant neoplasm, such as MM, whereas intermediate values of in vitro response rates were observed in BC, in agreement with clinical findings. Moreover, within each histologic subgroup in vitro sensitivities to individual drugs reproduced their clinical patterns of sensitivity.

Table 1. In vitro sensitivity of tumors with known different degrees of clinical chemosensitivity

| Drug | In vitro response rate (%) | | |
	NHL	BC	MM
4-OOH-Cyclophosphamide	63 (35)*	25 (25)	12 (8)
Doxorubicin	53 (102)	32 (74)	13 (30)
CCNU	43 (16)	7 (14)	14 (35)
Vinca alkloids[†]	26 (70)	18 (38)	16 (70)

* In parenthesis, number of tumors.
[†] Vincristine and vindesine.

Successively, the perspectives and limits in predicting individual tumor sensitivity were evaluated in three different ways. In vitro sensitivity to the drugs used in the preceding chemotherapy was analyzed in relation to the type of clinical response in a series of 64 tumors including NHL, EOC and GCTT (Table 2). A higher frequency of residual sensitivity to the drugs previously used was observed in tumors that relapsed after remission induction than in those that progressed during chemotherapy. An intermediate fraction of tumors still sensitive was observed in partial responders.

Table 2.   In vitro sensitivity in relation to clinical response to preceding chemotherapy

Clinical response	Tumor type	No. of tumors sensitive to at least one drug/no. of tumors tested	
Progression	NHL	3/5	
	GCTT	0/8	
	EOC	0/4	
Total			3/17* (17%)
Partial response	NHL	1/2	
	GCTT	4/12	
	EOC	4/8	
Total			9/22 (41%)
Relapse	NHL	10/17	
	GCTT	2/5	
	EOC	2/3	
Total			14/25* (56%)

* $p = 0.03$

In vitro sensitivity was also analyzed in relation to response to subsequent standard clinical treatment including the same drugs tested in vitro. An updating of the clinical correlations is reported in Table 3. In these series of patients clinical protocols consisted of cisplatinum, vinblastine or etoposide, and bleomycin regimens (PVB or PEB) for GCTT; cyclophosphamide, vincristine, doxorubicin (A), bleomycin, and prednisolone in different combinations (CVP∼ABP or BACOP) for NHL; doxorubicin and vincristine (AV) for BC; and different combinations of cyclophosphamide, doxorubicin and cisplatinum (CAP, CA, CP) for EOC. All the patients included in the analysis had advanced disease, and in vitro sensitivity was analyzed in relation to clinical objective response in terms of complete remission (CR) for GCTT and NHL, or CR plus partial response (PR) greater than 50% for BC and EOC.

From the overall analysis a significant agreement between in vitro and clinical results was observed in 79% of the cases (p=0.00003). Specifically, the true-positive and true-negative rates were respectively directly and inversely related to the clinical chemoresponsiveness. This study has also clearly shown the interlesional heterogeneity in drug sensitivity. In fact, in patients with GCTT there was very poor agreement between in vitro sensitivity of the primary tumor and clinical response of metastatic disease after orchidectomy; however, when the assay was performed on metastatic disease it predicted overall metastatic response in a high percentage of tumors (93%).

Table 3. Retrospective study: relationship between in vitro sensitivity and clinical response

Tumor type	No. of cases	Clinical response rate (%)	True-positive rate (%)*	True-negative rate (%)[+]	Overall agreement (%) [‡]	p value
GCTT						
Primary	17	94	100	14	65	NS
Metastasis	14	86	100	67	93	0.003
NHL	57	70	83	66	79	0.0003
BC	41	46	75	81	78	0.0001
EOC	20	10	40	100	85	0.01
Total	149	59	83	73	79	0.00003

* True-positive rate: (no. of sensitive both in vitro and in vivo/no. in vitro sensitive) x 100.
[+] True-negative rate: (no. of resistant both in vitro and in vivo/no. in vitro resistant) x 100.
[‡] Overall agreement: (no. of sensitive plus resistant both in vitro and in vivo/no. tested) x 100.
NS, not significant.

In a more recent study the results of the in vitro chemosensitivity assay were used to select clinical treatment in pretreated patients with advanced disease (Table 4). The in vitro assay was performed with drugs conventionally used for first-line or salvage standard clinical protocols for each tumor type. Drugs that were inactive in vitro were used for clinical treatment only when no blind chemotherapy was available. Clinical response was standard as CR in GCTT and NHL and as PR greater than 50% in EOC.

Table 4. Prospective clinical-aiding study: summing up of clinical predictivity

Tumor type	No. of cases	True positives*	True negatives[+]	P value
GCTT	15	4/7	8/8	0.01
NHL	7	4/6	1/1	NS[‡]
EOC	5	1/1	4/4	0.02
Total	27	9/14	13/13	0.0004

* True positives = no. sensitive in vitro and in vivo/no. in vitro sensitive.
[+] True negatives = no. resistant in vitro and in vivo/no. in vitro resistant.
[‡] NS, not significant.

A good predictivity of in vitro sensitivity on clinical response to tailored treatment was observed in the overall group. For NHL alone, in spite of the high overall agreement, the association between in vitro and clinical drug sensitivity was not statistically significant. In this series of tumors with a

poor clinical response, true-negative rates were very high in all tumor types
(100%), and true-positive rates were lower, as observed in the retrospective
study. In particular, in GCTT the use of in vitro-active drugs also allowed a
better long-term clinical outcome (Fig. 1). In fact, the probability of being
progression free at 7 months was 56% in patients treated with in vitro-active
drugs compared to 0% in those treated with inactive drugs (p=0.01).

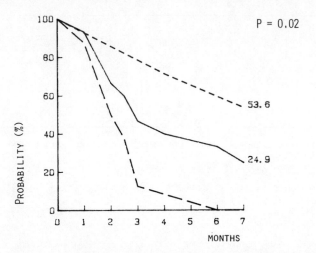

Fig. 1. Progression-free probability of patients with GCTT
         treated with in vitro active or inactive drugs.
         Inactive (— — —); active (- - -); overall (————).

APPLICATION OF THE NPI ASSAY TO BASIC STUDIES

An important application to the knowledge of the biology of drug-cell interaction in human tumors is the study of the relationships among the activities of
drugs similar or unrelated in structure and action mechanisms, for the analysis
of patterns of natural or induced cross-resistance. In particular, on the basis
of the knowledge of patterns of pleiotropic drug resistance in many animal and
human cell lines (Ling, 1982), the in vitro assay was used to verify the
occurrence of cross-resistance among anthracyclines, other antibiotics and vinca
alkaloids in human tumor biopsies (Table 5).

In vitro activities of doxorubicin and vincristine at clinically relevant
concentrations were compared in different tumor types; in testicular tumors the
study was enlarged to doxorubicin, actinomycin D and vinca alkaloids.   The
activities of doxorubicin and vincristine were differently associated in the
different tumor types with the highest association and a high coresistance rate
in BC, a trend to association in NHL, and no association in GCTT.   In the
latter, the two antibiotics as well as the two vinca alkaloids showed very
similar patterns of activity. In fact, high cosensitivity and even higher
coresistance rates were observed.

Another field of application deals with tumor heterogeneity. In vitro (Schlag,
1982; Sanfilippo, et al, 1983; Zaffaroni, et al, 1983; Tanigawa, et al, 1984)
and clinical (Berdeaux, et al, 1985) studies have shown different drug sensitivities not only among similar tumors but also among different tumor lesions of
the same patient. We used the short-term assay to analyze drug sensitivity
profiles of synchronous tumor lesions of the same patient. Conventional drugs

Table 5.   In vitro matched activities of similar or unrelated drugs at clinically relevant concentrations in different tumor types

| Drugs | Tumor type | No. of cases | Agreement rate (%) | | P |
			Cosensitivity*	Coresistance†	
Dx/Vc‡	GCTT	21	21	65	NS
	NHL	51	34	47	0.06
	BC	22	30	63	0.04
Dx/Ad	GCTT	26	40	73	0.03
Vc/Vb	GCTT	21	57	82	0.016

* (No. of tumors sensitive to both drugs/no. of tumors sensitive to at lease one drug) x 100.
† (No. of tumors resistant to both drugs/no. of tumors resistant to at lease one drug) x 100.
‡ Dx, doxorubicin; Vc, vincristine; Ad, actinomycin D; Vb, vinblastine.

with different action mechanisms, such as anthracyclines, other antibiotics, alkylating agents and vinca alkaloids, were tested in different tumor types, including BC, GCTT, EOC and CRC (Table 6). A significantly higher frequency of discordances in chemosensitivity was observed between the primary tumor and its metastasis than between different synchronous metastases (36% vs 15%, p=0.027).

Table 6.   Relationship of drug activities among different tumor lesions in the same patient

Tumor material	No. of tumors	Discordant one-drug tests/no. of tests
Primary vs metastasis	52	56/155
Synchronous metastases	9	5/34

DISCUSSION

Chief groups working with in vitro chemosensitivity tests have demonstrated the specificity of these models in reproducing the patterns of clinical sensitivity of different human tumor types.   The prediction of individual patients response to treatment analyzed by retrospective and prospective studies seems also to be satisfactory, even though the still limited number of patients, often hetero- geneous by risk factors, and the lack of randomized studies make it difficult to define the actual benefits and the cost—benefit ratio of a tailored therapy versus conventional trials.   Objective clinical limitations such as surgical inaccessibility or psychologic refusal of performing surgery other than for therapeutic purposes limit to only those patients with a poor prognosis the access to assay-directed clinical protocols.   Moreover, the natural or induced resistance of these advanced and/or previously treated tumors lessens the possi- bility to find active drugs.

However, clinical correlations reported in the literature have demonstrated the biologic reliability of these assays and their possible use also to investigate basic aspects related to testing of new drugs, drug resistance, and tumor heterogeneity on a system closer to clinical reality than experimental tumors or long-term human cell lines. The use of these assays seems to be promising for detecting resistant tumors. In fact, the possibility of analyzing the characteristics of resistance in large series of tumors with different clinical and biologic characteristics could make it possible to identify groups of patients with intrinsically resistant tumors.

Moreover, in the field in which we are presently involved, the possibility of studying human tumor biopsies makes it possible to verify the occurrence of some mechanisms of drug resistance known from experimental tumors, such as pleiotropic drug resistance. It is also possible to verify the heterogeneity in drug sensitivity or to simultaneously evaluate multiple cellular mechanisms of resistance such as inhibition of nucleic acid synthesis and pharmacokinetic parameters.

In conclusion, the experience accumulated in the last 10 years seems to substantiate the reliability of in vitro assays as intermediate systems between experimental tumors and in vivo human tumors for a better understanding of many aspects of drug-tumor interactions and as a preclinical means to easily and quickly define drug sensitivity.

ACKNOWLEDGMENTS

The authors thank Dr. E. Grignolio and Dr. C. Coltrocampi for assistance in the study, Miss C. De Marco and Miss R. Motta for technical assistance, and Ms. B. Johnston for editing and preparing the manuscript. The study was supported by Special Project "Oncology", contract numbers 84.00789.44 and 84.00808.44, from the Italian National Research Council, Rome.

REFERENCES

Berdeaux, D.H., T.E. Moon, and F.L. Meyokens Jr. (1985). Cancer Treat. Rep. 69, 397–401.

Bosanquet, A.G., M.C. Bird, W.J.P. Price, and E.D. Gilby (1983). Br. J. Cancer 47, 781–789.

Courtenay, V.D., P.J. Selby, I.E. Smith, J. Mills, and M.J. Peckham (1978). Br. J. Cancer 38, 77–81.

Daidone, M.G., R. Silvestrini, and O. Sanfilippo (1981). In: Adjuvant Therapy of Cancer, S.E. Salmon and S.E. Jones, eds., Grune & Stratton Inc., New York, pp. 25–32.

Daidone, M.G., O. Sanfilippo, N. Zaffaroni, and R. Silvestrini (1982). Proc. International Cancer Congress, Seattle, vol. 1915, p. 337.

Daidone, M.G., R. Silvestrini, O. Sanfilippo, N. Zaffaroni, M. Varini, and M. De Lena (1985). Cancer, 56, 450–456.

Dendy, P.P. (1981). Arch. Geschwulstforsch., 51/1, 111–118.

Durkin, W.J., U.K. Ghanta, C.M. Balch, D.W. Dorris, and R.N. Humamoto (1979). Cancer Res., 39, 402–407.

Hamburger A.W., and S.E. Salmon (1977). Science, 197, 461–463.

KSST (Group for sensitivity testing of human tumors) (1981). Cancer, 48, 2127–2135.

Ling, V. (1982). In: Drug and Hormone Resistance in Neoplasia, N. Bruchovsky and J.H. Goldie, eds., CRC Press Inc., Boca Raton, pp. 1–19.

Maddox, A.M., D.A. Johnston, B. Barlogie, M. Hag, M.J. Keating, and E.J. Freireich (1984). Eur. J. Cancer Clin. Oncol., 29, 507–514.

Morasca, L., E. Erba, M. Vaghi, C. Ghelandoni, C. Mangioni, C. Sessa, F. Landoni, and S. Garattini (1983). Br. J. Cancer, 48, 61–68.

Possinger, K., O. Wetlitzky, R. Hartenstein, and W. Wilmanns (1983). Proc. International Conference on Predictive Drug Testing on Human Tumor Cells, Zurich, 1983.

Preisler, H.D., J. Epstein, A. Raza, N. Azarnia, G. Browman, L. Booker, J. Goldberg, A. Gottlieb, J. Brennan, H. Grunwald, K. Rai, R. Vogler, L. Winton, K. Miller, and R. Larson (1984). Eur. J. Cancer Clin. Oncol., 29, 1061-1068.

Sanfilippo, O., M.G. Daidone, A. Costa, R. Canetta, and R. Silvestrini (1981). Eur. Eur. J. Cancer, 17, 217-226.

Sanfilippo, O., R. Silvestrini, N. Zaffaroni, and L. Piva (1983). Proc. ASCO, San Diego, C145, 37, Waverly Press, Inc., Baltimore.

Sanfilippo, O., M.G. Daidone, N. Zaffaroni, and R. Silvestrini (1984). In: Recent Results in Cancer Research, vol. 94, V. Hofmann and G. Martz, eds., Springer-Verlag, Berlin, Heidelberg, 127-139.

Schwarzmeier, J.D., E. Pajetta, K. Mittermeyer, and R. Pirker (1984). Cancer, 53, 390-395.

Schlag, P., and W. Schreml (1982). Cancer Res., 42, 4086-4089.

Silvestrini, R., O. Sanfilippo, and M.G. Daidone (1983). In: Human Tumour Drug Sensitivity Testing in Vitro, P.P. Dendy and B.T. Hill, eds., Academic Press, London, 281-290.

Silvestrini, R., O. Sanfilippo, M.G. Daidone, and N. Zaffaroni (1984). In: Recent Results in Cancer Research, V. Hofmann and G. Martz, eds., Springer Verlag, Berlin, Heidelberg, 140-149.

Silvestrini, R., M.G. Daidone, A. Costa, and O. Sanfilippo (1985). Eur. J. Cancer Clin. Oncol., 21, 371-378.

Sondak, V.K., C.A. Bertelsen, D.H. Kern, and D.L. Morton (1985). Cancer, 55, 1367-1371.

Tanigawa, N., Y. Mizuno, T. Hashimura, K. Honda, K. Satomura, Y. Hikasa, O. Niwa, T. Sugahara, O. Yoshida, D.H. Kern, and D.L. Morton (1984). Cancer Res., 44, 2309-2312.

Thomas, D.G.T., J.L. Darling, E.A. Paul, T.J. Mott, J.N. Godlee, J.S. Tobias, L.G. Capra, C.D. Collins, C. Mooney, T. Bozek, G.P. Finn, S.O. Arigbabu, D.E. Bullard, N. Shannon and R.I. Freshney (1985). Br. J. Cancer, 51, 525-532.

Tisman, G., V. Herbert, and H. Edlis (1973). Cancer Chemother. Rep., 57, 11-19.

Volm, M., K. Wayss, M. Kaufmann, and J. Mattern (1979). Eur. J. Cancer, 15, 983-993.

Weisenthal, L.M., J.A. Marsden, P.L. Dill, and C.K. Macaluso (1983). Cancer Res., 43, 749-757.

Wheeler, T., P. Dendy, and A. Dawson (1974). Oncology, 30, 362-376.

Zaffaroni, N., R. Silvestrini, O. Sanfilippo, M.G. Daidone, and C. De Marco (1983). Proc. 13th International Congress on Chemotherapy, K.H. Spitzy and K. Karrer, eds., Verlag H. Egermann, Vienna, vol. 11, pp. 143-146.

Biological and Pharmacological Considerations for Human Tumor Clonogenic Cell Studies

M. S. Aapro

Division of Oncology, University Hospital,
1211 Geneva 4, Switzerland

ABSTRACT

In spite of some promising results for predictive drug testing, clonogenic
cell assays need careful definition of the conditions in which they are used.
Inter-laboratory variations make quality control mandatory. Better growth of
clonogenic cells can be obtained by various means, some of which might modify
drug testing. Assay systems using only defined media are to be preferred. A
linear relationship between plated cell concentration and colony number is not
always observed. The influence of medium and cells themselves on the
cytotoxic activity of a drug can be important. Drug stability and mode of
action are among others factors that need to be taken into account.
Clonogenic cell assays are not limited to drug testing and their major role is
in the study of tumor biology.

KEYWORDS

In vitro growth; clonogenic; colony; drug testing; prognosis; cytotoxic drug.

INTRODUCTION

Growth of hemopoietic cells in semi-solid media has allowed substantial
advances in our understanding of the development of both normal and abnormal
blood cells (Metcalf, 1977). Human tumor clonogenic cells can be studied with
several methods (Hamburger and Salmon, 1977, Courtenay et al, 1978, and
others). Chemosensitivity testing of fresh human tumor clonogenic cells has
been studied by many groups. In a compilation of 635 trials, Salmon (1984)
reports a 71% true-positive and a 91% true-negative rate for predicting drug
sensitivity and resistance, respectively, of cancer patients to chemotherapy.
Such predictions might have an important clinical impact, as it has been
suggested that relapsing ovarian cancer patients might have an improved
survival when treated according to in vitro data (Alberts and Surwit, 1981).

IMPORTANCE OF QUALITY CONTROL

Even though many groups using clonogenic assays have reported that they can
confidently predict sensitivity or resistance to antitumou agents, any centre
wishing to use such methods should first validate its own results by a
correlative trial. As it is true for any biological assay, modifications of
cell growth or drug testing conditions can influence observed results. The

EORTC Clonogenic Assay Screening Study Group (Rozencweig, 1983) reported its
first study on inter-laboratory reproducibility of in vitro drug sensitivity
testing using clonogenic assays in 1985. We observed major problems with
variations in growth of a colon cell line (WiDr) and with reproducibility of
some drug sensitivity testing results. Since then, a second study (to be
published) has shown that intensive exchange of information and
standardization of some procedures can solve many problems. Our group has
decided to continue checking each member laboratory's growth conditions at
least twice a year. Similar results have been obtained by other groups
(Leudke et al, 1984; Clark et al, 1984) and should be reviewed as quite
encouraging, as the overall reproducibility of drug sensitivity or resistance
data is satisfactory.

POOR GROWTH

However, testing chemosensitivity of fresh human tumor samples in a clonogenic
assay is a frustrating experience. In most laboratories less than half of the
samples will grow sufficiently to allow any evaluation. Reasons for such poor
growth and, generally, low plating efficiencies, lie in the unsatisfactory
semi-solid media and growth conditions, and in the nature of the plated cells
themselves.

IMPROVING GROWTH CONDITIONS

Considerable efforts have been made to obtain better plating efficiencies.
Use of enzymatic rather than mechanical dissociation might be helpful (Slocum
et al, 1981; Besch et al, 1983; Engelholm et al, 1985) but the influence of
enzymes on membrane integrity and drug sensitivity has not been sufficiently
addressed. Then, centrifugation through a density-gradient like Ficoll could
be used to remove unwanted debris and dead cells (Gaines et al, 1983; Katoh et
all, 1984). Many other important technicalities, like quality of agar
(Thomson et al, 1983) can influence growth. Low oxygen content of incubators
might be crucial. It has dramatic influence on growth of melanoma cells
(Tveit et al, 1981) and is standard for the Courtenay assay. Addition of more
undefined elements to the "Hamburg and Salmon" assay, for example cell-free
ascities (Uitendaal et al, 1983) or tumor-cell conditioned media (Hug et al,
1984) has been advocated. We, and others, have used a different approach and
tried to obtain a better defined medium (Eliason et al, 1984; Carney et al,
1983). Using an entirely defined complex medium first developed for the study
of hemopoietic progenitor cells in methylcculose, we have been able to reduce
serum content to 5 percent. However, studies of hormmones or other biological
modifiers will need serum-free media. Further improvements of all proposed
media should be forthcoming, and, for example, the role of epidermal growth
factor remains to be defined (Pathak et al, 1984). It is probable that
different histological tumor types, and different malignant cells n the same
tumor, have diverse needs for in vitro growth.

BIOLOGICAL MEANING OF "NO GROWTH"

Even with the best in vitro growth conditions, some tumor cells will grow
poorly, or not at all. I have recently reviewed the expanding body of
evidence that gives some biological meaning to this phenomenon (Aapro, 1985).
For bladder, breast, head and neck and ovarian cancer, there seems to be a
relation between good prognosis and lack of in vitro growth. It is quite
possible that only the most malignant, ie, most metastasizing, cells can grow
in our artificial systems. Further studies will have to clarify the
relationship between cell ploidy, labelling index, metastasizing capacity,
laminin receptors and other factors with growth of colonies in semi-solid
media. Patient's characteristics and tumor stage will hve to be considered as
they may sometimes complicate correlations of laboratory and clinical data.
Obviously, once tumor burden is too important, some prognostic factors can
become useless.

NON LINEARITY OF COLONY FORMATION

When colonies do grow, it ;is important to know if there is a linear
relationship between the concentration of cells plated and the colony number.
We have recently observed that in 23 samples examined, only 9 appeared to be
linear (Eliason et al, 1985). Eight samples had an increasing cloning
efficiency with increasing cell concentration and in 6 the cloning efficiency
was less at the highest cell concentrations than at lower cell
concentrations. These results indicated that clonogenic assays with fresh
tumor materials are not necessarily linear. Similar observations have been
made by other authors (Meyskenss et al, 1983). Modulation of in vitro growth
by cooperativity between cells and lack of some nutrients in the media can
both explain these observations. They provide a clue to apparent stimulation
of in vitro growth by cytotoxic agents and can also explain some of the
discrepancies between the tumor's in vitro and in vivo behaviour. If an
efficacious inhibitor agent is tested in vitro, it will decrease the number of
colony forming cells. Wehn the clonogenic assay used is non-linear, such a
decrease can be reflected by a paradoxal increase or a tremendous decrease in
the number of colonies formed. Figure 1 shows how this can be understood when
thinking at the reciprocal statement, that which is usually observed : colony
growth. If the assay is non linear, a decrease in colony number from 2 y to y
can be a decrease in viable progenitor cells from 2x to 1.6x or from 2x to
0.3x. We propose that at least 3 cell concentrations should be used in
control plates, particular when cytotoxic drugs are tested in vitro.

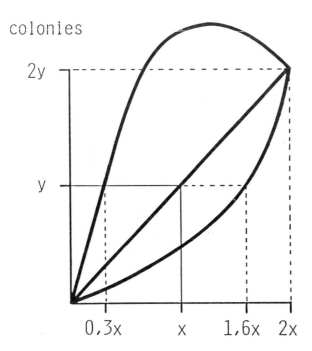

Figure 1.   Relation of progenitor cell number (x) to colony number (y) when
                      assays are non-linear.

TESTING SINGLE DRUGS THAT ARE ACTIVE IN VITRO

The stability of cytotoxic drugs after dissolution and short or long-term
conservation in frozen aliquotes has been the object of contradictory reports
(Franco et al, 1984; Ludwig and Alberts, 1984; Yang and Drewinko, 1985). It
thus seems advisable that, unless one can afford to make a fresh preparation
daily, each laboratory should verify its own storage conditions of drugs. It
is on purpose that I have not included a table showing how each author
prepared his stock solution. The concentration of drug used for
chemosensitivity testing in clonogenic cell assays has been proposed to be
one-tenth of the clinically achievable plasma levels (Alberts et al, 1981).
Higher concentrations would possibly improve the accuracy for prediction of
resistance but sensitivity would be over-predicted. Duration of exposure of
cells to drugs is another variable. One-hour exposure might not always be
adequate, for example for cell-cycle phase specific agents (Rupniak et al,
1983), but most "predictive" studies have been used such a length of
exposure. Again, as stated above, each laboratory should define its own
"predictive" conditions in a prospective (or retrospective) study. Finally
some cytotoxic agents are inactive in vitro, as they have to be metabolized
(eg, cyclophosphamide) (Lieber et al, 1981).

Little attention has been paid to the importance of the medium in which cells
are exposed to drugs. Some agents, like methotrexate or cisplatin, bind
strongly to proteins and their in vitro activity can be considerably modified
in a medium containing 2.5% human serum albumin (Inoue et al, 1984). Similar
decreases of in vitro toxicity has been observed for other agents (Aapro
et al, 1984; Daniels et al, 1984). We have also studied the effect of cell
concentration and observed, (like Herve et al, 1983; Arkin et al, 1984), a
marked decrease in the cytotoxic effect of several drugs when target cell
concentrations are increased (figure 2).

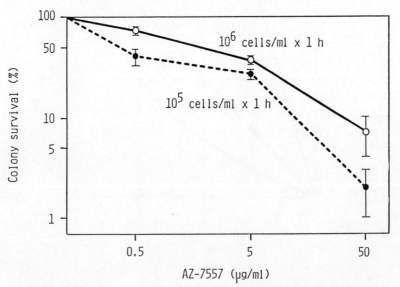

Figure 2.   Cell line: 8226.   Influence of Nucleated Cell Concentration.

Thus, two major problem areas have been recently identified and the impact of these observations on the clinical use of clonogenic cell assays is evident. These observations are crucial when one is contemplating the use of cytotoxic or other drugs for bone-marrow purging before autologous transplantation, as that is a situation in which considerable quantities of cells are manipulated in various types of media.

CONCLUSION

This paper was not intended to be a comprehensive review of in vitro drug testing using clonogenic assays. Other authors in this book have addressed other drug-testing systems and also discussed drug combination testing. Many important contributations to the field have been overlooked. While one has to realise that predictive drug testing with the use of clonogenic assays is quite difficult, one has also to understand that these systems are remarkable tools for the study of tumor biology, from karyotypic anomalies (Trent et al, 1980), to mechanisms of cellular cooperation (Hamburger and White, 1982).

ACKNOWLEDGEMENTS

The Geneva and Swiss Cancer Leagues, the Swiss National Science Foundation have supported our studies mentioned in this paper. I would like to express my gratitude to all colleagues, technicians and secretaries for their constant cooperation and advice.

REFERENCES

Aapro, M., M. Brink-Peterson, V. Roosens and P. Alberto (1984). Proc. AACR, 25, 331.
Aapro, M. (1985). Eur. J. Cancer Clin. Oncol., 21, 397-400.
Alberts, D.S., S.E. Salmon, H.S.G. Chen, T.E. Moon, L. Young and E.A. Surwit (1981). Cancer Chemother. Pharmacol., 6, 153-264.
Alberts, D.S. and E.A. Surwit (1981). Proc. 13th Int. Cancer Congress, Seattle, p. 78, and personal communication (updated data) 1983.
Arkin, H.R. Ohnuma, J.F. Holland and S.D. Gailani (1984). Proc. AACR, 25, 315.
Besch, G.J., W.H. Wolberg, K.W. Gilchrist, J.G. Voelkel and M.N. Gould (1983). Breast Cancer Res. Treat., 3, 15-22.
Calvo, F., D.N. Carney, M. Browner and J.D. Minna (1983). Br. J. Cancer, 48, 683-688.
Carney, D.N., A.F. Gazdar and J.D. Minna (1982). Proc. Am. Soc. Clin. Oncol., 1, 10.
Clark, G.M. and D.D. von Hoff (1984). In: Human Tumor Cloning, Eds Salmon S.E. and Trent J.M., Grune & Stratton, Orlando, FL., 255.
Courtenay, V.D., P.J. Selby, I.E. Smith, J. Mills and M.J. Peckham (1978). Brit. J. Cancer, 38, 77-81.
Daniels, A.M. and Daniels J.R. (1984). Proc. AACR, 25, 376.
Eliason, J.F., A. Fekete, and N. Odartchenko (1984). Rec. Res. Cancer Res., 94, 267.
Eliason, J.F., M.S. Aapro, D. Decreyl and M. Brink-Petersen (1985). Proc. AACR, 26, 364.
Engelholm, S.A., M. Spring-Thomsen, N. Brünner, I. Nohr and L.L. Vindelov (1985). Br. Cancer, 51, 93-98.
Franco, R., T. Kraft, T. Mille, M. Popp and O. Martelo (1984). Int. J. Cell Cloning, 2, 2-8.
Gaines, J.T., C.E. Welander and H.D. Homesley (1983). Proc. AACR, 24, 331.
Hamburger, A.W. and C.P. White (1982). Stem-Cells, 1, 209-223.
Hamburger, A.W. and S.E. Salmon (1977). Science, 197, 461-463.
Herve, P., E. Manayo and A. Peters (1983). Br. J. Haematol., 53, 683-690.
Hug, V., M. Haynes, R. Rashid, G. Spitzer, G. Buemenschen and G. Hortobagyi (1984). Br. J. Cancer, 50, 207-213.
Inoue, S., T. Ohnuma, T. Okano, J.F. Holland and O.S. Selawry (1984). Proc. AACR, 25, 320.

Katoh, A.K., S. Charoensiri, P. Fogarty and C. Best (1984). Arch. Pathol. Lab. Med., 108, 305-307.

Lieber, M.M., A.M. Ames, G. Powis and J.S. Kovach (1981). Life Sci., 28, 287-293.

Ludwig, R. and D.S. Alberts (1984). Cancer Chemother. Pharmacol., 12, 142-145.

Luedke, D.W., F.J. Carey, A. Krishan, D. Chee, B. Chang, R. Franco, H.B. Niell, M.E. Johns, D.E. Kenady and K. Zirvi (1984). In: Human Tumor Cloning, Eds Salmon S.E. and Trent J.M., Grune & Stratton, Orlando, Fl., 245.

Metcalf, D. (1977). In: Hemopoietic colonies: in vitro cloning of normal and Leukemic cells, Springer-Verlag, Berlin.

Meyshens, F.L. Jr., S.P. Thomson, R.A. Hicke and J.J. Sipes (1983). Br. J. Cancer, 48, 863-868.

Pathak, M.A., L.M. Matrisian, B.E. Magun and S.E. Salmon (1982). Int. J. Cancer, 30, 745-750.

Rozencweig, M. (1983). Proc. AACR, 24, 313.

Rupniak, H.T., R.D.H. Whelan and B.T. Hill (1983). Int. J. Cancer, 32, 7-12.

Salmon, S.E. (1984). Cancer Treat. Rep., 68, 117-125.

Slocum, H.K., Z.P. Paveli, A.M. Rustum, P.J. Creaven, C. Karakousis, H. Takita and W.R. Greco (1981). Cancer Res. 41, 1428-1434.

Thomson, S.P., M.D. Wright and F.L. Meyskens Jr. (1983). Int. J. Cell Coning, 1, 85-91.

Trent, J.M. and S.E. Salmon (1980). Cancer Genet. Cytogenet., 1, 291-296.

Treit, K.M., L. Endresen, H.E. Rugstad, O. Fodstad and A. Phil (1981). Brit. J. Cancer, 44, 539-544.

Uitendaal, M.P., H.A.J.M. Hubers, J.G. McVie and H.M. Pinedo (1983). Br. J. Cancer, 48, 55-59.

Yang, L.Y. and B Drewinko (1985). Cancer Res., 45, 1511-1515.

PART TWO

TOPICS IN NEURO-ONCOLOGY

Biological Correlates of Brain Tumor Pathology

D. Schiffer

The 2nd Neurological Clinic, University of Turin, Italy

ABSTRACT

The problem of anaplasia is discussed in relation to the possibility of demonstrating the loss of differentiation. Some demonstratio-
ns are given by immunohistochemistry applied to astrocytic gliomas.

KEYWORDS

Anaplasia; gliomas; immunohistochemistry.

Anaplasia is the main problem of astrocytic gliomas. Classically,
it is regarded as the consequence of dedifferentiation, that is the
loss of morphological characteristics, typical of a degree of cell
differentiation, with regression to characteristics of a more primitive stage. However, it can be also conceived as the failure of
differentiation: the cells do not reach morphological maturation
(Zimmerman, 1962). As a consequence, not only glioblastoma, but also typical immature tumors, such as medulloblastoma, can be called
anaplastic. The only difference remains cell atypia, present in the
former and not in the latter. As a matter of fact, it is not easy
to define anaplasia especially if the term is referred not to the
tissue but to the cells. The meaning could be different according
to whether the cells are considered anaplastic in comparison to
their normal counterparts or in comparison to their parent cells.
In recent years anaplasia is being regarded more and more as the
product of heterogeneity of tumor cell population. This has been
established on the ground of kariotypic (Mark et al.1977; Shapiro and
Shapiro,1981), cytophotometric, flow cytometric (Hoshino et al.
1979; Hoshino,1984) analyses and comparisons among established cell
lines of human gliomas (Bigner et al.1981). However, whether changes of phenotype are produced by genetic variations, due to the

77

progressive increase of mutation rates of tumor cell populations,
or by epigenetic factors, such as those outlined by Duffy (1983),
is still debated (Bigner,1981; Rubinstein et al.1984).
The question is not simply academical, because in the epigenetic
hypothesis a cell property might disappear and reappear according
to a modulation, regulated by enviromental factors. In the other
hypothesis the disappearance of a cell character could have very
few statistical probabilities of being followed by its reappearance. This ambiguity in the conception of anaplasia shows up chiefly
when applied to the problem of differentiation-dedifferentiation of
astrocytic gliomas.
This problem has been studied by investigating immunohistochemically the GFAP expression in different areas of glioblastomas and
astrocytomas, (Schiffer et al. submitted) corresponding,to the microenvironments outlined by Shapiro and Shapiro (1984). GFAP has
been assumed as a typical example of a cell characteristic of differentiation (see for reviews De Armond and Eng, 1984 and Bonnin
and Rubinstein, 1984). Also Vimentin has been immunohistochemically
studied (Schiffer et al. submitted), because this intermediate fi-
lament in embryonic life is expressed much earlier than GFAP
(Schnitzer et al.1981; Bignami et al.1982; Pixley and De Vellis,
1984) and therefore can be regarded as a cell characteristic of im-
maturity.
Either the appearance of anaplasia in astrocytoma or of actively
proliferating populations in glioblastomas are given by cells with
scanty cytoplasm, lacking GFAP expression and with many mitoses.
In glioblastomas they represent most cells of invasive and proliferative areas, whereas in central areas GFAP-positive cells prevail.
If mitoses are evaluated for GFAP expression, it can be found that
GFAP-negative districts are very rich in mitoses which are GFAP-negative; districts mostly GFAP-positive are poor in mitoses which
are mostly GFAP-positive and mixed districts show an intermediate
number of mitoses which are mostly GFAP-negative. It can be deduced
that we are dealing with two cell populations showing different
growing velocities.

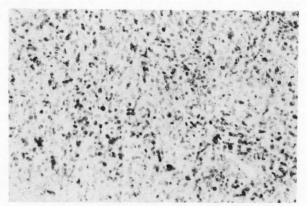

Fig.1.Invasive area of glioblastoma:small,GFAP-negative cells,200x

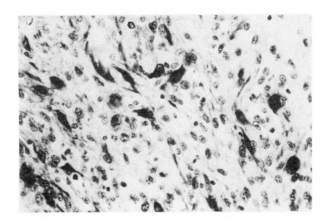

Fig.2. Central area of glioblastoma:many large cells are GFAP-positive, 300 x.

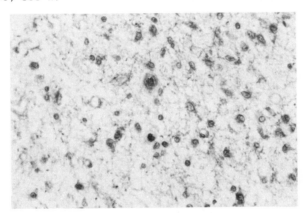

Fig.3. Glioblastoma:GFAP-positive and -negative mitoses, 300 x.

The distribution of Vimentin in gliomas repeats that of GFAP,with
a lower reaction intensity. Besides endothelial and mesenchymal
cells, Vimentin decorates ependymal cells and in astrocytic gliomas
those cells which are intensely GFAP-positive. These observations
are different from those made by others (Yung et al.1985) and do
not seem to support the conclusion that tumoral glia is immature
because Vimentin-positive. Both types of intermediate filaments
seem undergo in the cells the same occurrences and both are strongly positive in reactive astrocytes. The variation of their expression in gliomas does not fit with the antinomy immaturity-differen-
tiation till now regarded as the biological basis for the interpretation of the pathology of gliomas and especially of their maligni-
zation.

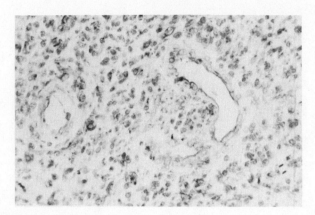

Fig.4. Glioblastoma: positive reaction for vimentin in tumor and
endothelial cells, 300 x.

In undifferentiated tumors the appearance of a glial differentiation with GFAP expression is a quite common phenomenon (Rubinstein
et al.1984; Feigin et al.1983; Roessmann et al.1983), as it can be
easily observed in PNET (Hart and Earle,1973). However, the problem
we are dealing with is more complicated. It would be very interesting to know whether the new anaplastic population composed of
GFAP-negative cells could give rise to GFAP-positive cells in the
long run or not. In other words the problem is if differentiation
could follow dedifferentiation. The question is closely related to
the occurrence of astrocytomatous areas in glioblastomas. Since the
actively proliferating subpopulations must gain selective advantage
on the other population for the progression of the tumor (Schmitt,
1983; Rubinstein et al.1984) the answer should be negative.
Obviously, the effects of environmental factors on the expression
of intermediate filaments must not be underestimated. Giant cells
of glioblastomas, which cannot reproduce (Hoshino et al.1972), may
be both GFAP-positive and negative and this must be attributed to
enviromental factors.
Two other points deserve to be emphasized: the role played by reactive astrocytes in the tumor growth and the biological significance
of circumscribed necroses with pseudo-palisadings. Reactive astrocytes which develop around the tumors are intensely GFAP-positive
and show long and thick processes and sometimes mitoses. Their nucleus is large and vesiculous. When they get trapped in the advan-
cing tumor proliferation, they lose processes and are no longer
distinguishable from GFAP-positive tumor astrocytes, not even for
the GFAP-positive mitoses which occur in both cell populations.
What could be the role they play in the morphological composition,
if not in the proliferation, of peripheral tumor areas is not
known.From the immunological point of view they seem to play an

active role (De Tribolet et al.1984). There is no doubt that their occurrence in peripherally located areas may be, at least, misleading, because a GFAP-positive reaction might be attributed to an actively proliferating population which, on the contrary, is negative.
Circumscribed necroses with pseudo-palisadings have been already regarded by us as expression of rapid growth (Schiffer et al.1982). This consideration has been confirmed from the clinical and prognostic point of view (Nelson et al.1983). They develop from centres of active growth in the tumor as the final product of a mitotic imbalance (Waggener and Beggs,1976) since the mean generation time of endothelial cells is longer than that of tumor cells (Tannock,1971), so that necrosis is realized through an inadequate vascularization. They are surrounded by many mitoses and contain inside lymphocyte-like nuclei which are constituted, as already demonstrated by us (Schiffer et al.1966), of denaturated DNA and represent mitoses from which nuclei do not recover.
Circumscribed necroses are found mainly in peripheral invasive areas where many reactive astrocytes, intensely GFAP-positive, may occur. The astrocytes do not seem to react to necrosis or to accumulate around it, but rather to undergo passively the occurrence. In fact they may go involved and be damaged by the necrosis. Maybe the rapidity with which they respond is lower than that with which necroses develop from proliferative centres.
In conclusion, old concepts, such as anaplasia, to-day hardly comprehensible from the morphological point of view, must be revised and new bases must be found.

ACKNOWLEDGEMENT
Supported by a grant of the Italian National Research Council, Special Project "Oncology", contract number 84.00796.44. and by the Italian Association for Cancer Research (A.I.R.C.)

REFERENCES
Bigner, D.D., Bigner, S.H., Pontèn J., Westermark, B., Mahaley, M.S., and E. Rouslahti, et al. (1981). J. Neuropathol. Exp. Neurol. 40, 201-229.
Bigner, D.D. (1981). Neurosurg. 9 320-326.
Bonnin, J.M., and L.J. Rubinstein (1984). J. Neurosurg. 60, 1121-1133.
De Armond, S.J. and L.F. Eng (1984). Progr. exp. Tumor Res. 27, 92-117.
De Tribolet, N., Piguet, V., Diserens, A.C., Mach, J.P., and S. Carrel (1984). In: Caciagli, F., Giacobini, E., and R. Paoletti. Developmental Neuroscience: Physiological, Pharmacological, and Clinical Aspects, Elsevier, Amsterdam, 20, 273-279.
Duffy, P.E. (1983). Astrocytes: normal, reactive and neoplastic,

Raven Press, New York.

Feigin, I., Epstein, F., and J. Mangiardi (1983). J. Neuro-oncol. 1, 95-108.

Hart, M.N., and K.M. Earle (1973). Cancer 32, 890-897.

Hoshino, T., Barker, M., Wilson, C.B., Boldrey E.B., and D. Fewer (1972). J. Neurosurg. 37, 15-26.

Hoshino, T., and C.B. Wilson (1979). Cancer 44, 956-962.

Hoshino, T. (1984). Progr. exp. Tumor Res. 27, 83-91.

Mark, J., Westermark, B., Pontèn, J., and R. Hugosson (1977). Hereditas 87, 243-260.

Nelson, J.S., Tsukada, Y., Schoenfeld D., Fulling, K., Lamarche,J., and N. Peress (1983). Cancer 52,550-554.

Roessmann, U., Velasco M.E., Gambetti P., and L. Autilio-Gambetti (1983). J. Neuropathol. exp. Neurol. 42, 113-121.

Rubinstein, L.J., Herman M.M., and S.R. Vanderberg (1984). Progr. exp. Tumor Res. 27, 32-48.

Schiffer, D., Fabiani, A., Monticone, G.F., and A. Cognazzo (1966). Acta Neuropathol. (Berlin) 6, 290.

Schiffer, D., Giordana, M.T., Soffietti R., and R. Sciolla (1982). Acta Neuropathol. (Berlin) 58, 291-299.

Schiffer, D., Giordana M.T., Mauro, A., and I. Germano (1985). In press.

Schiffer, D., Giordana M.T., Mauro, A., Migheli, A., Germano I., and G. Giaccone (1985). In press.

Schmitt, H.P. (1983). Path. Res. Pract. 176, 313-323.

Shapiro, J.R., Yung, W.A., and W.R. Shapiro (1981). Cancer 41, 2349-2359.

Shapiro, J.R. and W.R. Shapiro (1984). Progr. exp. Tumor Res. 27, 49-66.

Tannock, I.F. (1970). Cancer 30, 2470-2476.

Zimmerman, H.M. (1962). In: Fields._W.S., and P.C. Sharkey.The biology and treatment of intracranial tumors, Thomas, Springfield.

Waggener, J.D., and J.L. Beggs (1976). In: Thompson, R.A., and J.R. Green. Neoplasia in the Central nervous system, Raven Press, New York, 15, 27-51.

Brain Tumor Stem Cells: Influence of Different Culture Conditions

M. L. Rosenblum, D. A. Emma,
H. Kleppe-Hoifodt, D. V. Dougherty, J. Giblin,
J. T. Rutka and M. A. Gerosa

Brain Tumor Research Center, Department of Neurosurgery,
University of California, San Francisco, USA

INTRODUCTION

The human organism and all its functional components originate from stem cells with the ability to reproduce itself(self-renew). During growth and the development of the specific organ systems, the number of differentiated cells increases. The normal human bone is an example of such a cellular hierarchy. Within bone marrow there is a progressive transition of undifferentiated cells with maximal self-renewal capability, through partially differentiated cells with some ability to self renew, to terminally differentiated cell systems. Local environmental influences that modulate the cellular traverse through the hierarchy include: the state of oxygenation and nutrition, the presence of growth factors (colony-stimulating factors), associations with non-hematopoietic cells present in the bone marrow, and the bone marrow matrix.
Tumors are also generally considered to originate from a single stem cell, which, for some reason, is no longer totally modulated by its local environment. Chemicals, viruses, irradiation and spontaneous mutations are thought to alter the cell at the DNA level and serve as the initial event in oncogenesis. Recent discoveries on oncogenes and their role in tumor induction, promotion and progression, have provided a biochemical bridge between these DNA events and eventual malignant transformation. Particularly intriguing is the observation of specific oncogene amplification and/or alterations with attendant secretion of growth factors and the presence of growth factor receptors.

It is presumed that an understanding of stem cell biology is necessary to best comprehend tumor growth and to develop means of curing, rather than merely palliating patients with malignant brain tumors. Unfortunately, at the present time, we are not able to unequivocally identify all the stem cells within any solid tumor. As a consequence, <u>in vitro</u> methods have been developed to grow and study tumor cells that can

operationally be defined as stem cells; the definition is based on a cell's
proliferative capacity to divide 4-7 times and develop into a colony
containing 16-128 cells. It is most correct to refer to such colony forming
cells as "clonogenic", rather than 'stem', in order to signify the potential
problems attendant with in vitro isolation and quantitation of this self-
renewing population.
Clonogenic cells will develop into colonies in an anchorage-dependent
fashion in monolayer culture   and in an anchorage-independent fashion
using soft-gel matrix systems. We have evaluated the colony forming
efficiency (CFE) of tumor cultures using monolayer, Courtenay, and
Hamburger-Salmon (H-S) assays.

METHODS AND RESULTS

        The standard monolayer (1), Hamburger-Salmon (2), and Courtenay
(3) techniques were used with five cell lines derived from malignant gliomas
(SF-126, SF188, SF-268, A-2781, U-251 MG). Table 1 outlines the CFEs for
these three assays performed on the five tumors and shows that the CFE in
monolayer was always greater than that in either the Hamburger-Salmon or
the Courtenay assays.
Cultures were plated for growth inthe monolayer system and cells were
harvested at various times for subsequent plating for colony formation using
the Courtenay assay. The plating efficiency appeared to increase dramati-
cally from the early exponential to the exponential phase and then decrease
as the cells reached the confluent contact-inhibited phase (unpublished
observations).
        Six tumor cultures were evaluated for the addition of a variety
of medium additions to the 10% fetal calf serum-MEM medium that has been
routinely utilized for CFE studies of human malignant brain tumors (1).
We noted that six additions appeared to be stimulatory, and six inhibitory
when added to the basal medium. The method for evaluating stimulation or
inhibition   was incorporation of tritiated thymidine using a microtiter well
system with a Titer-Tek Analysis System.

TABLE 1   Colony Forming Efficiency (CFE) for standard
             clonogenic cell assays.

Tumor No.	Mean CFE (%)		
	Monolayer	Hamburger-Salmon	Courtenay
SF-126	33.5	1.0	3.0
SF-188	8.2	1.3	7.5
SF-268	5.4	3.1	15.4
A-2781	>95.0	23.0	38.1
U-251 MG	64.4	2.3	1.6

In decreasing order of stimulation the following additions were noted to improve tritiated thymidine incorporation and, bv presumption. monolayer cell proliferation: putrescine, PGE-1, bovine serum albumin (BSA), non essential amino-acids, aminoguanidine (a polyamine-oxydase inhibitor), and dexamethasone.
The following factors appear to be inhibitory in a decreasing order of growth inhibition: DEAE Dextran. cholesterol. tryptic soy broth, sodium pyruvate. calcium chloride, and mercaptoethanol. There was no significant effect on growth with ascorbic acid. asparagine, gentamycin, glucose, glutamine, hydrocortisone, insulin, selenium, serine. tocopherol. or transferrin (unpublished observations).
The effect of the growth stimulating factors on clonogenic assays were determined by adding the following growth stimulating factors to the Courtenay assay using three cell lines: putrescine, PGE-1, BSA. and dexamethasone. The colony forming efficiency was increased in one of the three tumors utilized (SF-210, but not SF-268 or SF-188).
The colony size however, was increased both in SF-210 and SF-188.
We evaluated the elimination of inhibiting factors (tryptic soy broth, DEAE Dextran, 2-mercaptoethanol, ascorbic acid. insulin, and L-serine) from the Hamburger-Salmon system. using four cell lines developed in our laboratory; we noticed that elimination of the inhibitors increased the plating efficiency of tumor cells 2-to 26-fold. This increase in plating efficiency was observed in both the 20% oxygen environment as well as in the 5% oxygen environment.
Finally, we noted that a 5% oxygen environment increased the colony forming efficiency in the Hamburger-Salmon assay in all three cell-lines tested. There appeared to be less of an effect of the 5% oxygen environment using the Courtenay assay in comparison to the 20% oxygen environment (unpublished observations). The addition of August rat red blood cells increased the plating efficiency in four out of six experiments in the 5% oxygen athmosphere. There was no significant overall difference noted with the addition of red blood cells using 20% ambient oxygen.

CONCLUSIONS

The CFE in monolayer was always greater than in agar.
Growth in the Courtenay assay was usually better than in Hamburger-Salmon systems. Furthermore, the state of proliferation of cells prior to plating for colony formation, medium-constituants. and the environmental oxygen concentration influenced the CFE.
Therefore, it is apparent that the cells we define as clonogenic will depend upon the culture conditions employed. As a consequence, conclusions derived from biochemical and molecular biological studies of the clonogenic cell population might differ from one laboratory to another.

REFERENCES

1. *Rosenblum M.L., Vasquez D.A., Hoshino T., Wilson C.B. (1978). Cancer 41 : 2305-2314.*

2. *Hamburger A.W., Salmon S.E. (1977). Science 197: 461-463.*

3. *Courtenay V.D., Selby P.J., Smith I.E., Mills J., Peckham M.J. (1978) Br. J. Cancer 38: 77-81.*

Production of BCNU-resistant 9L Brain Tumor Cells *in vivo* and *in vitro*

M. L. Rosenblum* and M. A. Gerosa**

*Brain Tumor Research Center, University of California
San Francisco, San Francisco, USA
**Department of Neurosurgery, University of
Verona, Verona, Italy

ABSTRACT

A clonogenic cell assay developed for the 9L rat brain tumor model was used to
investigate the production of tumor cell resistance to 1,3-bis (2-chloroethyl)-
1-nitrosourea (BCNU). The BCNU dose-response curve obtained from the solid
tumor treated in vivo showed exponential cell kill with a plateau at 3 to 4 logs,
a plateau that was not observed after in vitro treatment of cultured 9L cells.
By contrast, in vitro treatment of cells derived from the solid tumor confirmed
the same plateau as a result of the survival of BCNU-resistant cells.
Twenty cultures were obtained from cells surviving various doses of this
nitrosourea either in vivo or in vitro. The development and the degree of BCNU-
resistance were shown to be related to the drug-dose used prior to cell
harvesting . Furthermore, highly BCNU-resistant cell lines were found to be
stable over 28 culture passages.
Finally, markedly resistant cells were obtained at a lower level of cell kill
in vivo than in vitro. This differential production of BCNU-resistant cells is
probably due to either intercellular interactions within the solid tumor or to
other host factors.

KEY WORDS

Stem cell; clonogenic cell; BCNU; drug-resistance; brain tumor.

INTRODUCTION

A colony-formation assay was developed in our laboratory to determine the in
vitro clonogenic capacity of cells in an experimental rat brain tumor (9L gliosarcoma) (12). The comparison of the colony-forming-efficiency (CFE) of cells
taken from 9L gliosarcoma growing in untreated rats and in rats treated with
chemotherapeutic agents proved to be a sensitive, reliable, quantitative measure
of in vivo tumor cell kill (10,11,14). Similar encouraging results have been
obtained with the human brain tumor clonogenic cell assay (8,9,13).
Therefore, this approach was considered a suitable method for investigating the
development of tumor cell resistance to nitrosoureas both in vivo and in vitro.
The present studies describe the production of BCNU-resistant cell cultures
following single dose BCNU treatment of 9L brain tumors growing and treated in
vivo, as well as cultures growing and treated in vitro.
A panel of BCNU-resistant cells have been developed which should serve as a
model system to investigate the mechanism(s) of resistance to this drug.

87

MATERIALS AND METHODS

In vivo Production of Resistant Cells.
Fisher 344 rats bearing 9L brain tumors were treated intraperitoneally with
single doses of 0.5 to 2.0xLD_{10} (6.7 to 26.7 mg/kg) of BCNU. All rats were
sacrificed 24 hr. later; the tumors were immediately removed, weighed, minced,
and disaggregated to single cells by a 30 min. exposure to an enzyme cocktail
(DNAse, pronase, collagenase) according to a method described previously (8,
12-14). Aliquots of the single cell suspensions were used to determine tumor
cell kill by CFE analysis (10,13,14).
Another group of rats with 9L tumors were similarly treated with a 1 or 2xLD_{10}
(13.3 or 26.6 mg/kg) dose of BCNU. After 24 hr., the tumors were disaggregated
and the clonogenic cells assayed. Surviving cells were passaged in culture to
develop larger cell populations. Subsequently, some of these previously drug-
exposed cells were challenged in vitro with single or several doses of BCNU
and cytotoxicity was evaluated by CFE analysis. Another portion of cells
surviving in vivo BCNU treatment was implanted intracerebrally into a second
group of rats. The solid tumors that subsequently developed were treated
in vivo with an LD_{10} dose of BCNU. In vivo chemosensitivity was analyzed by
CFE assay, as well as by simultaneous animal survival studies. In all instances,
untreated tumor-bearing rats served as control.
In vitro Production of Resistant Cells.
Aliquots of 9L cells growing in culture flasks with the complete medium (10-12)
were treated in vitro with graded, single doses (3 to 21 ug/ml x 1 hr.) of BCNU.
Cells were removed by trypsinization after 1 hr. of exposure to the drug, and
immediately replanted in 60 mm. Petri dishes and in large culture flasks for
CFE analysis. Clonogenic cells surviving treatment with the 8,10 and 14 ug/ml
dosages were again treated in vitro with 8 ug/ml of BCNU and then processed for
the CFE assay.
Stability of Resistant Cells in Culture.
Cells were harvested from tumors treated in vivo with 2xLD_{10} dose of BCNU,
tested for BCNU sensitivity using the CFE assay, and frozen in liquid N_2 for
later analysis. Cultures of BCNU-resistant cells were thawed 4 years later, and
passaged weekly with a split ratio of 1:2/1:4. Cell survival analyses were
performed on serial culture passages to determine the stability of BCNU -
resistance in the 9L model system.

RESULTS AND DISCUSSION

Analysis of BCNU Resistance.
BCNU sensitivity was analyzed using the stem cell assay, and a comparison was
made between cells surviving the initial in vivo and in vitro drug treatments.
The cell survival curve for 9L gliosarcomas treated in vivo with BCNU (Fig. 1a)
was similar to the curves obtained in previous studies (10-12,14): exponential
cell kill increased up to 3-4 logs at 13.3 mg/kg (1xLD_{10}); beyond this dosage
level, there was no further cell kill.
In contrast, the cell survival curve derived after in vitro treatment of cells
from 9L cultures (Fig. 1b) initially had a small shoulder region and then
showed exponential cell kill to approximately 5 logs at 9 ug/ml.
Although there was additional cell kill noted at 14 ug/ml, the slope was less
steep and possibly represents the initial portion of a plateau.
The plateau on the in vivo dose-response curve of intracerebral tumors could be

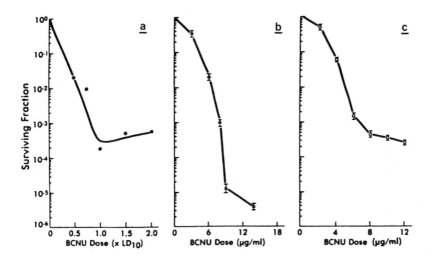

Fig. 1 - Analysis of BCNU resistance using the CFE assay.

1a. The survival curve of clonogenic cells, harvested from 9L rat brain tumors 24 hr after _in vivo_ treatment with various doses of BCNU ($1xLD_{10}$ = 13.3 mg/kg), shows exponential cell kill with a plateau at 3-4 log kill at $1xLD_{10}$ dose or greater. Each point represents an individual tumor; the curve was drawn by best eye-fit.

1b. The surviving fraction of clonogenic 9L rat brain tumor cells was determined for _in vitro_ cultures that were treated with various doses of BCNU (3-14 ug/ml x 1 hr). Exponential cell kill was observed to the level of approximately 5 log kill; the error bars represent standard errors.

1c. Single cells were disaggregated from solid brain tumors that had not been exposed to therapy _in vivo_; 48 hr later, these _in vivo_-derived cells were treated _in vitro_ with various doses of BCNU (2-12 ug/ml x 1 hr). The dose-response curve has a shape that is similar to the curve derived from _in vivo_ treatment of solid tumors, with a plateau at 3 to 4 log cell kill. The error bars represent standard errors.

TABLE 1   In vivo and in vitro production of BCNU-resistant tumor cell lines

| | First Treatment | | | In vitro (8ug/ml) | | | Second Treatment In vivo (13.3mg/kg) | | | | |
| | | | | Log Kill[1] | | | Log Kill[1] | | ILS(%)[3] | | |
Mode	Dose	Culture N.	Log Kill[1]	CTRL	SURV	R[2]	CTRL SURV		CTRL SURV		R[2]
In Vivo	2xLD$_{10}$	1	3.42	1.80	0.39	marked	2.48 0.62		95	2	marked
	(27mg/kg)	2	3.36	2.98	0.40	marked			42	0	marked
		3	3.04	2.98	0.64	marked					
		4	3.36	2.98	0.52	marked					
		5	3.39	2.98	0.71	marked					
		6	3.74	1.96	0.59	marked	2.79 1.71		61	5	mod. to marked
	1xLD$_{10}$	7	2.96	2.40	1.24	moderate					
	(13.3mg/kg)	8	3.00	2.40	1.27	moderate					
		9	2.81								
		10	2.88								
		pool 7-10	2.91	1.66	1.34	slight	2.61 2.40		75	50	slight
		pool 11-14	2.62	2.33	1.34	moderate					
		pool 15-17	3.28	2.24	2.24	none	2.46 3.02		54	53	none
In Vitro	14ug/ml	18	5.40	3.92	2.11	moderate					
	10ug/ml	19	n.a.	3.22	3.22	none					
	8ug/ml	20	3.00	3.00	3.72	none					

1 Log Kill= The negative log of the surviving fraction, as determined by the ratio between the CFE of the treated and the CFE of the untreated cells (11-14). The log kill noted for pooled cells that had received their first treatment in vivo is the mean of the log kills for each of the tumors pooled. The log kill recorded for the second treatment in vivo is the mean value for tumors from 3 rats treated in both control and pretreated groups. CTRL=controls; SURV=survivors.

2 R=BCNU resistance determined according to the ratio between Log Kill Controls/Log Kill Survivors. R was arbitrarily defined as marked (ratio > 1.8), moderate (1.4-1.8), slight (1.2-1.4), or none (<1.2).

3 ILS= Increased life span of treated rats (in %) as compared to nontreated rats, with groups of > 10 rats in all groups.

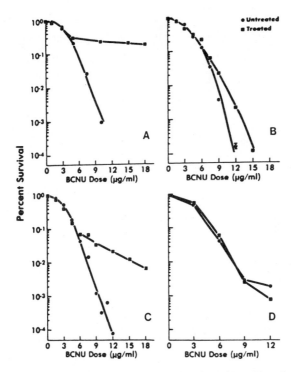

Fig. 2 - In vitro BCNU dose-response curves for four 9L cell cultures (3/4 pooled) that had survived in vivo administration of an LD_{10} (13.3 mg/kg). The four graphs represent four separate series of experiments (see TABLE 1). The symbols indicate the surviving fraction of clonogenic cells after treatment with various BCNU concentrations (2-18 ug/ml x 1 hr); the standard error never exceeded 10% of the mean value for the SF. Several experiments were performed using equal numbers of tumor cells pooled from different tumors that had been exposed in vivo to an LD_{10} dose; in vitro analyses were performed immediately after the pooling of cells. The squares (■) represent the pretreated cells; the circles (●) represent untreated control cells.

2A. Marked BCNU resistance was demonstrated for tumor culture $9L_6$.
2B. Slight resistance for cells pooled from $9L_7$- $9L_{10}$.
2C. Moderate resistance for cells pooled from $9L_{11}$- $9L_{14}$.
2D. No resistance for cells pooled from $9L_{15}$-$9L_{17}$.

the result either of inadequate drug delivery to all cells within the solid
tumor or of the presence of BCNU-resistant cells. In order to investigate
which of these factors might be responsible for the plateau, cells from the
untreated solid 9L tumor that had been used in the in vivo experiments noted
above (Fig. 1a) were disaggregated to single cells and within 48 hr treated with
graded doses of BCNU (2 to 12 uM) in vitro (Fig. 1c).

The in vitro dose-response curve for these dissociated cells was similar to the
curve derived after the in vivo treatment of 9L tumor: exponential cell kill
was observed up to 3-4 logs at a dosage level of 9 ug/ml BCNU; with higher doses
there was a plateau. We therefore concluded that the plateau on the in vivo
BCNU dose-response curve is probably the result of the survival of BCNU-resistant
cells.

Several BCNU-resistant cell lines were developed by treating both solid tumors
and cell cultures with single, large doses of BCNU (TABLE 1); the cell lines
were not cloned for this study. Cells surviving in vivo administration of 26.7
mg/kg BCNU were markedly resistant to the drug in 6/6 tumors tested, whereas
cells surviving an in vivo dose of 13.3 mg/kg showed responses ranging from
marked resistance to marked sensitivity to BCNU (TABLE 1; Fig 2). In three
cases, equal numbers of cells were pooled from 3 or 4 tumors immediately before
in vitro or in vivo analysis of BCNU resistance. The slight or moderate BCNU
resistance observed in the pooled cell populations could have been caused by the
presence of significant numbers of resistant cells in one or more of the pooled
tumors; however, the observation of no resistance in the pooled population
implies that none of the pooled tumors contained a significant number of resistant cells under the conditions of our assay. It appeared that the degree of
resistance was related to the in vivo BCNU dosage, even though surviving cells
at all dosage levels were either near or on the plateau of the cell-survival
curve.

In contrast to the in vivo treatment studies, cells surviving an in vitro BCNU
dosage of 8 or 10 ug/ml (approximately 3 log cell kill) were sensitive to BCNU,
and cells surviving 14 ug/ml in vitro -5.4 log cell kill) were only moderately
resistant to BCNU (see TABLE 1).

Resistance Stability

Repeated in vitro analyses of one of the most resistant 9L cell lines ($9L_1$)
confirmed that BCNU resistance was stable after the cells had been frozen for
as long as 4 years, as well as after cells had undergone 28 culture passages
over a period of 6 months (Fig. 3).

The growth rate of several BCNU-resistant cell lines was the same or slightly
slower, both in vivo and in vitro, than the growth rate of the sensitive cells
(unpublished observations).

CONCLUSIONS

It is generally thought that phenotypic drug-resistance may be inherent in a
tumor cell population, and that it may become evident only after the sensitive
cells have been eliminated by effective therapy (2,7,15,18).

Mathematical models have been used to estimate the rate of spontaneous mutation
of clonogenic tumor cells to their drug-resistant phenotype (6,16,18,19).
Alternatively, however, resistance may develop as a result of the administration
of X-rays, ultraviolet radiation, carcinogens or chemotherapeutic agents (1,4,
20). This "induction" of resistance may occur as a consequence of alterations

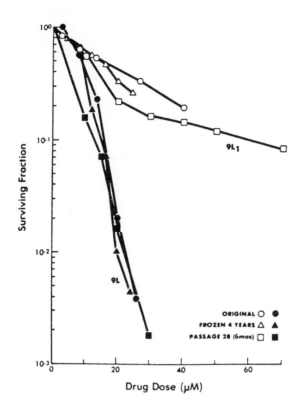

Fig. 3 - Analysis of the stability of BCNU-resistance in 9L₁

The graph summarizes three different series of experiments: the dose-response curves on the original 9L and 9L₁ lines (● ○), on the same two cell lines thawed and planted after having been frozen for four years in liquid nitrogen (▲ △), and finally, after 28 culture passages over 6 months (■ □).
Symbols represent the mean Surviving Fraction of clonogenic cells at different doses of BCNU, expressed as uM x hr exposure doses.
The standard errors never exceeded 10% of the mean value.
The marked resistance of 9L₁ cells to BCNU treatment <u>in vitro</u> appears stable over the period studied and not significantly altered by frozen storage techniques.

in cellular metabolism - the stability of this "induced" resistance is a controversial issue- (1,4,5,17,20), or as a result of an increased mutation rate to
the resistant phenotype, catalyzed by an applied mutagen: a classic example of
the latter mechanism is the induction of 8-azaguanine resistance in the Chinese
Hamster cell line V79-379 A by two anthracene derivatives (3).

Our preliminary experiments suggest that BCNU resistance occurs with higher
frequency after BCNU treatment in vivo than in vitro, despite there being
equivalent levels of cell kill in both conditions. This might indicate that the
rate of spontaneous or host-induced mutation to BCNU resistance in vivo ($>10^{-4}$)
is different from that in vitro ($<10^{-5}$) (16,17).

In contrast to tumor cells in the in vitro environment, which are dissociated
from one another and are individually exposed to the chemotherapeutic agent,
cells within the solid tumor coexist in intimate relation with one another and
in association with normal host cells, such as macrophages and immunocompetent
cells. It appears that some mechanism unique to the in vivo environment is
responsible for the increased expression of cellular resistance to BCNU in vivo.
Further investigations are under way to clarify the molecular mechanism of BCNU
resistance and its possible genetic implications.

ACKNOWLEDGEMENTS

        We are indebted to Dr. Enrico Mihich, Director of the Department of
Experimental Therapeutics and Grace Cancer Drug Center, Roswell Park Memorial
Institute,Buffalo, New York; and to George Stark, Professor of Biochemistry,
Stanford University, for reviewing this work and for their very helpful sugge-
stions. We thank Susan Eastwood for editorial assistance, and Beverly McGehee
for preparation of the manuscript. This work was supported by grants CA-13525,
CA-31882, and CA-28529A1 from the National Institute of Health.
M.L.R. is the recipient of Teacher Investigator Development Award 1K07 NS 00604
from the National Institute of Neurological and Communicative Diseases and
Stroke, National Institute of Health, U.S.A.

REFERENCES

1. Anderson D., Fox M. (1974). Mutation Res. 25: 107-122.
2. Burchenal J.H. (1976). Cancer 37: 46-57.
3. Duncan M.E., Brookes P. (1974). Mutation Res. 26: 37-48.
4. Fox M. (1974). Mutation Res. 23: 129-145.
5. Friedrich U., Coffino P. (1977). Proc. Natl. Acad. Sci. (U.S.A.) 74:679-683.
6. Goldie J.H., Coldman A.J. (1979). Cancer Treat. Rep. 63: 1727-1733.
7. Norton L., Simon R. (1977). Cancer Treat. Rep. 61: 1307-1317.
8. Rosenblum M.L. (1980). In 'Cloning of Human Tumor Stem Cells', S.E. Salmon ed. pp. 259-276, Alan Liss Co., New York.
9. Rosenblum M.L., Gerosa M.A., Wilson C.B., Barger G.R., Pertuiset B.F., De Tribolet N., Dougherty D.V. (1983). J. Neurosurg. 58: 170-176.
10. Rosenblum M.L., Knebel K.T., Vasquez D.A., Wilson C.B. (1977). J. Neurosurg. 46 : 145-154.
11. Rosenblum M.L., Knebel K.T., Vasquez D.A., Wilson C.B. (1976). Cancer Res.36: 3718-3725.
12. Rosenblum M.L., Knebel K.T., Wheeler K.T., Barker M., Wilson C.B. (1975). In Vitro 11: 264-273.
13. Rosenblum M.L., Vasquez D.A., Hoshino T., Wilson C.B. (1978). Cancer 41: 2305-2314.
14. Rosenblum M.L., Wheeler K.T., Wilson C.B., Barker M., Knebel K.T. (1975). Cancer Res. 35: 1387-1391.
15. Salmon S.E. (1979). In 'Adjuvant Therapy of Cancer. II', Jones S.E. & Salmon S.E. eds., pp. 27-36, Grune-Stratton Publ., New York.
16. Skipper H.E. (1980). Monograph Series from Southern Research Institute, Booklets I-17, pp. 1-45, Birmingham, Alabama.
17. Skipper H.E., Hutchinson D.J., Schabel F.M., Schmidt L.H., Goldin A., Brockman R.W., Venditti J.M., Wodinski I. (1972). Cancer Chemother. Rep. 56: 493-498.
18. Steel G.G., Lamberton L.F. (1968). Natl. Cancer Inst. Monogr. 30: 29-50.
19. Swan G.W. (1977). In 'Some Current Mathematical Topics in Cancer Research' 1-6 pp. 71-83, University Microfilm International, Ann Arbor, Michigan.
20. Taylor R.T., Carver J.H., Hanna M.L., Wandres D.L. (1979). Mutation Res. 67 : 65-80.

Antiglioma Monoclonal Antibodies

E. Frank and N. de Tribolet

Service de Neurochirurgie, CHUV, 1011 Lausanne, Switzerland

Key words: Glioma   Monoclonal Antibody   Brain Tumor   Antigens

INTRODUCTION

A major breakthrough in immunology occurred in 1975 with the development of the technology for the production of monoclonal antibodies (Köhler and Milstein, 1975). This technique utilizes the fusion of nonspecific antibody secreting myeloma cells with naturally occurring specific antibody secreting spleen cells. The somatic cell hybrids produced in this fusion codominantly express immortality and specific antibody production, so that the transient property of specific antibody secretion can be fixed as a permanent property of an established cell line.

With the advent of the MAB, the quest to identify specific antigens on the surface of glioma cells advanced rapidly. The initial search for these antigens was slow. Polyclonal antibodies were produced either from autologous sera of glioma patients or from heterosera of animals immunized with extracts of human gliomas (Coakham, 1975, 1984-1, Mahaley, 1972, Martin-Achard et al, 1980, Pfreundschuh et al, 1978, Schnegg et al, 1981, Wikstrand et al, 1977). These antisera required prolonged absorption on normal tissues in order to remove contaminating non glioma antibodies. When this process was completed, very small quantities of antibody remained for study.

Using MAB two major groups of antigens present on glioma cells have been identified. The first group of antigens found on glioma cells, the tumor associated antigens includes the neuroectdermal antigens and the glioma antigens. The neuroectodermal antigens have a fairly wide representation on neuroectodermal tumors, but may be used in a novel way for immunolocalization of gliomas. In contrast, the glioma antigens are present on glial cells and dendritic cells of the thymus, spleen and liver and may be used advantageously for immunohistological diagnosis.

The second group of antigens identified are lymphoid differentiation antigens which play an important role in cellular immune function. The presence of these antigens on glioma cells and adjacent endothelial cells suggests that cells within the central nervous system might have some immune functions.

In this review we will discuss the different groups of antigens found on glioma cells, the relationship of these antigens to the host immune response and the means by which MAB raised against these antigens might be employed for diagnosis, localization and therapy of malignant gliomas.

TUMOR ASSOCIATED ANTIGENS

Neuroectodermal antigens constitute a major component of the surface antigens found on glioma cells. They are also present on other tissues and tumors derived from the neuroectoderm. In vivo, these antigens have been detected on melanomas, neuroblastomas, gliomas, as well as fetal brain cells and endothelial cells within gliomas (Cairncross et al, 1982, Carrel et al, 1982-1, Dickinson et al, 1983, Kennett et al, 1978, Piguet et al, 1985, Seeger et al, 1981). Screening with MAB for these antigens has demonstrated that there is no common neuroectodermal antigen on neuroectodermally derived tissues. These tissues and tumors express these antigens singly or in groups.

The detection of melanoma antigens on the endothelia of vessels within malignant gliomas is an interesting phenomenon (Schreyer et al, 1985). The presence of these antigens on tumor cells attests their neuroectodermal origin while the expression of the same antigen on the endothelial cells suggests that some transformation has taken place in antigenic representation. The expression of the melanoma antigens on tumor vasculature might provide a sophisticated method for localization of gliomas.

Glial antigens are primarily present on gliomas and have some additional minor specificity for other non neuro ectodermal tissues and reactive astrocytes Bourdon et al, 1983, de Tribolet, 1980, de Tribolet et al, 1984). The overall representation of these antigens on human gliomas has been studied using panels of MAB (de Muralt et al, 1983).

Several important concepts emerge from the studies of glioma antigen representation. First, MAB are produced from glioma cells that have been grown in vitro. Since cells grown in this manner have changes in their surface antigen expression, it is necessary that all MAB be evaluated immunohistologically in vivo. Second, tumor antigens are not present on all the cells of a given glioma. Third, the actual antigenic determinants recognised by some MAB may be present on some totally unexpected cells of normal tissues. This stresses the necessity of thoroughly screening the MAB before using them in vivo.

Finally, it has become evident that a glioma is not a homogeneous collection of cells all having the same antigenic determinants. Actually, the cells of a glioma have a constantly varying multiprobable antigenicity (Bigner, 1982, Bourdon et al, 1983, Shapiro et al, 1981, Wikstrand et al, 1983). Many intrinsic and extrinsic factors can alter or induce changes in cellular antigen expression. Factors such as cell age, state of each cell in its cell cycle, heterogeneity of the original clonogenic cells, external humoral factors, external immune interactions and the effects of attempted therapy could all affect antigen expression. This antigenic variability limits the probability that a single antigen would be resident on all or even a critical number of glioma cells at one time. Therefore the possibility that a single MAB could direct therapy would be low. Perhaps for such a therapy to be successful an artificially created poly-monoclonal antibody would be required in order to identify a critical number of tumor cells.

LYMPHOID DIFFERENTIATION ANTIGENS

The lymphoid differentiation antigens comprise a large group of antigens

expressed on systemic circulating lymphocytes. Included are lymphoid antigens
of functioning lymphocytes (Thy 1), antigens expressed by lymphocytes that have
undergone malignant change (CALLA) and antigens of the major histocompatibility
complex (MHC, eg. HLA-DR) (Carrel et al, 1982-2, Kemshead et al, 1982,
Seeger et al, 1982, Wikstrand et al, 1983). The recognition of these
antigens on cells of malignant gliomas has provided a unique view of the
existence and function of the immune system within the central nervous system
and gliomas in particular.

IMMUNOBIOLOGY OF THE HOST-GLIOMA INTERACTION

The expression of certain MHC antigens, particularly the Class II antigens HLA-
DR, is necessary for the initiation of a cellular immune response to a foreign
antigen. As a key step, HLA-DR must be displayed by the antigen presenting
cells so that they can present foreign antigen to helper T lymphocytes (Unanue
et al, 1984). The necessity for coexpression of Class II antigens and foreign
antigen on these cells forms a possible double check system to guard against
indiscriminate activation of T lymphocytes to normal antigens.

The second step in this response is that the T lymphocytes, once activated,
secrete lymphokines including interferon gamma (IFN gamma) and Interleukin 2
(IL2). IFN gamma serves as a feed foreward positive stimulus for antigen
presenting cells. HLA-DR expression is increased therefore enhancing further
foreign antigen presentation to lymphocytes. IL2 stimulates proliferation of
lymphocyte clones and helps activate the humoral immune response. The
elaboration of these two lymphokines by the T lymphocytes both enhances and
amplifies the immune system's recognition, processing and response to foreign
antigen.

It has been a surprise to find that activated astrocytes and glioma cells as
well as endothelial cells within the CNS have the ability to express HLA-DR and
that this expression is modulated by IFN gamma (Gerosa et al, 1984, Piguet
et al, 1985). The exact significance of this finding is unknown but it is
tempting to hypothesize that normal astrocytes within the CNS and glioma cells
may be able to function as antigen presenting cells when they express HLA-DR.
This idea is supported by the recent demonstration of rat astrocytic
presentation of myelin basic protein antigen to activate T lymphocytes in
vitro (Fontana et al, 1984-2).

All of this evidence refutes the concept that the CNS is an immunologically
privileged site and suggests that the CNS contains some cells that, if
provoked, may function as integral parts of the immune system.

One can develop a theoretical model of the host glioma interaction given the
above information. The glioma is a dynamic mass of malignant cells surrounded
by reactive astrocytes and pierced by abnormal vasculature. At any point in
time, some of the glioma cells will express glioma und neuroectodermal
antigens. The control of this antigen expression resting upon a combination of
intrinsic cellular mechanisms and extrinsic host factors. Endothelial cells of
the vascular structures coursing through and around the glioma may also express
lymphoid differentiation antigens and tumor associated antigens of the
neuroectodermal type. The presence of these antigens on the endothelial cells
signals their response to the nearby glioma, the mechanism of this being
unknown.

The cellular and humoral immune responses of the patient harboring a malignant
glioma are abnormal. While it was originally thought that this occurred because
the brain was isolated from the immune system, this may not be true. As

discussed above, astrocytes and some glioma cells may actually participate in the immune response. The presence of HLA-DR on the surfaces of these cells, in specific circumstances, and the knowledge that this expression can be influenced by IFN gamma hints that the potential for an active specific immune response exists.

To establish an immune response, the reactive astrocytes and the glioma cells bearing HLA-DR might interact with the infiltrating lymphocytes that are known to be present within gliomas. These astrocytes and glioma cells might present foreign glioma antigen to these lymphocytes, release Interleukin I (IL1), stimulate B lymphocyte as well as T lymphocyte clonal expansion and be further stimulated by the IFN gamma released by the activated lymphocytes. The endothelial cells within the glioma may also interact with the lymphocytic population. When the endothelia display HLA-DR, they might serve as the primary antigen presenting cells, presenting foreign antigen to immune cells in the systemic circulation and recruiting their diapedesis into the CNS.

This simplistic view of the immune response within a glioma is incomplete. At present we know that a glioma produces a factor that blocks the effects of IL1 and IL2 (Fontana et al, 1984-1).

This factor limits the IL1 effect on presentation of foreign antigen and the IL2 dependent expansion of lymphocytic clones. Both of these processes being necessary for sustainance of an active immune response. The glioma cells also secrete an additional factor which coats the cell wall and hinders direct interaction of glioma cells with other cells (Gately et al, 1982).

With this concept of the immunobiology of the malignant glioma in mind, how can this system be manipulated so as to more easily identify, localize and treat these malignant tumors?

IMMUNOHISTOLOGICAL DIAGNOSIS OF BRAIN TUMORS WITH MAB

With the development of MAB for glial and neuroectodermal antigens, techniques for immunohistological diagnosis of gliomas and other brain tumors have advanced rapidly. As a supplement to established histological techniques, the evaluation of tissue specimens with techniques employing MAB has expanded our ability to accurately identify specific groups of cells comprising brain tumors. Coakham and Brownell have been particularly keen in using MAB for this purpose. By this means they have established antigenetic profiles for many CNS tumors including meningiomas, gliomas, schwannomas, meduloblastomas and neuroblastomas (Coakham et al, 1984-2, 1985).

One important area in which immunohistological diagnosis is of particular importance is the analysis of small tissue specimens obtained by stereotactic biopsy. Accurate MAB assisted diagnosis of these biopsies may enhance selectivity in application of specific forms of therapy. Currently, our laboratory is analysing stereotactic biopsies with a panel of MAB. We have found that this technique greatly assists in the rapid diagnosis of cerebral gliomas and other tumors including metastasis.

IMMUNOLOCALIZATION OF GLIOMAS USING MAB

As an extension of the use of MAB for immunohistology, one might use systematically administered labelled MAB for in vivo immunolocalization. From the clinical standpoint, the in vivo ability for localization of gliomas, for the evaluation of their surgical removal and for the early detection of their recurrence would be extremely useful.

The MAB used for any _in vivo_ application must be carefully evaluated. The antigen binding to the MAB must be isolated and characterized, the affinity of the MAB for this antigen must be determined and the recognition of similar antigenetic determinants on normal tissue must be understood. The patients' reaction to foreign MAB protein and to the attached label must also be examined. Only with this information can a MAB be chosen that will be safe for the patient and will have the highest probability to locate and bind with the glioma antigen.

The blood brain barrier (BBB) retards the penetration of large molecular weight compounds into the CNS and therefore may limit the access of labelled MAB to glioma cells (Rapoport, 1975). This may not be a problem in the central necrotic areas of tumor where the BBB is abnormal either as a result of tumor induced vascular changes or to the necrosis of the vessels themselves. In this area large molecules could easily accumulate or pool. If this is the case then the presence of a labelled MAB could be nonspecific and result in false localization.

At the actively growing peripheral areas of tumor and in the brain adjacent to the tumor, the BBB is probably near normal as glioma cell growth appears to precede the development of abnormal vasculature. Identification of this area is of obvious importance for precise delineation of tumor size and or extension. Because of the problem with the BBB in this area, it might be necessary to utilize techniques of BBB disruption to enhance the penetration of labeled MAB (Neuwelt, 1984).

One form of immunolocalization that is attractive and presents fewer technical problems is the detection of neuroectodermal melanoma antigens on the vasculature within a glioma. Since the endothelial cells appear to express these antigens in response to tumor, one might be able to identify these antigens with labeled MAB and hence identify the tumor. This technique would not require that the labeled MAB cross the BBB or traverse the intercellular space to reach the glioma cells. Further investigation of the spatial and temporal expression of melanoma antigens on tumor vasculature is necessary before this technique can be studied clinically.

IMMUNOTHERAPEUTIC CONSIDERATIONS

Immunotherapeutic intervention might be possible at several levels. A MAB might be used as a carrier for chemotherapeutic or radiotherapeutic agents. The cellular immune system might be altered either by administration of exogenous lymphokines or by cloned activated lymphocytic cells. And lastly, one might try to overcome the effects of the blocking factors secreted by the glioma cells.

The possibility for using MAB as a carrier for therapeutic agents has been considered for many years but its realization has been slow. In order for MAB directed therapy to be safe, the antigens must be characterized and their representation on normal tissues must be minimal as stated above. Even if this was not a problem, there is always the possibility of an anaphylactic reaction to the foreign MAB protein particularly if the MAB is administered repeatedly.

Other problems that temper ones enthusiasm include the difficulty to link a MAB with a chemotherapeutic or radiotherapeutic agent without destroying either the specificity and affinity of the MAB or the toxic characteristics of the noxious agent and the penetration of the complex through the BBB. One must also recognise the multiprobable antigenitic variability of glioma cells as mentioned above.

Manipulation of the cell mediated immune response is another potential means of immunotherapy. The administration of IFN gamma could be a major stimulus for the cellular immune response within the CNS. IFN gamma penetrating into the area of the tumor would stimulate HLA-DR expression on the astrocytes and glioma cells. Knowing that similar cells are capable of presenting foreign antigen in an in vitro system, one could surmise that in vivo cells might act similarly after IFN gamma exposure. If a critical amount of antigen could be presented in this manner then an immune response might be initiated. This interaction might be further enhanced by coadministration of IL2 which would stimulate the expression of its own receptor on T lymphocytes and expand populations of lymphocytes and natural killer cells within the proximity of the tumor.

While this appears a logical way to stimulate the cellular events we must appreciate that the glioma cells are producing factors that block the interaction of IL1 and IL2 with T lymphocytes and also a mucopolysaccaride cell coat that limits recognition and presentation of foreign glioma antigen regardless of the expression of HLA-DR. The blocking factor to IL2 would also limit the amplification of the cellular immune response.

The problems posed by these blocking factors might be overcome with administration of an antibody to the factor. This might prove helpful with the factor that blocks IL1 and IL2 effetcs, but would have no efficacy against the encompassing cell coat.

The local or systemic administration of specifically activated autologous lymphocytes is another possible form of immunotherapy. Depending upon the actual type of lymphocytes infused, one of two reactions might occur: T lymphocytes could be cytotoxic to the tumor cells or they could play the pivotal role of helper T lymphocytes and coordinate T and B lymphocyte responses. Current state of the art techniques allow the expansion of selected lymphocyte clones activated by tumor cells and stimulated by IL2.

Several initial experiments using autologous cytotoxic T lymphocytes in a mouse model have proven to be encouraging (Yamasaki et al, 1984).

CONCLUSION

In this review we have discussed how antiglioma MAB have been used to identify and isolate specific groups of antigens expressed by malignant glioma cells. The recognition of these antigens and the development of these MAB have prompted the conceptualization and attempted creation of sophisticated methods for immunolocalization, immunodiagnosis and immunotherapy. As yet, only the ability to use these MAB for immunodiagnostic purposes has started to be commonly employed. Many problems must be dealt with before these MAB may be used for in vivo applications.

With the recognition of lymphoid differentiation antigens on glioma cells and astrocytes, we have gained a new perspective on the function of the immune system within the CNS. With this knowledge we can begin to think of ways that this immune reaction can be manipulated in order to limit the growth and development of intracerebral gliomas.

REFERENCES

Bigner, D.D. (1982). Neurosurg., 9, 320-326.
Bourdon, M.A. Wikstrand, C.J., Furthmayr, H., Matthews, T.J., and D.D. Bigner (1983), Cancer Res., 43, 2796-2805.

Cairncross, J.G., Mattes, M.J., Beresford, H.R., Albino, A.P., Houghton, A.N.,
Lloyd, K.O., and L.J. Old (1982). Proc. Natl. Acad. Sci., 79,
5641-5645.
Carrel, S., de Tribolet, N., and J.P. Mach (1982-1). Acta. Neuropath., 57,
158-164.
Carrel, S., de Tribolet, N., and N. Gross (1982-2). Eur. J. Immunol., 12,
354-357.
Coakham, H.B., and M.S. Lakshmi (1975). Oncology, 31, 233-243.
Coakham, H.B. (1984-1). Eur. J. Cancer Clin. Oncol., 20, 145-149.
Coakham, H.B., Garson, J.A., Brownell, B., and J.T. Kemshead (1984-2).
J. Royal Soc. Med., 77, 780-787.
Coakham, H.B., Garson, J.A., Allan, P.A., Harper, E.I., Brownell, B.,
Kemshead, J.T., E.B. Lane (1985). J. Clin. Path. 38, 165-173.
de Muralt, B., de Tribolet, N., Diserens, A.C., Carrel, S., and J.P. Mach
(1983). Anticancer Res., 3, 1-6.
de Tribolet, N., and S. Carel (1980). Cancer Immun. Immunotherapy 9, 207.
de Tribolet, N., Carrel, S., and J.P. Mach (1984). Prog. Exp. Tumor Res.,
27, 118-131.

Dickinson, J.G., Flanigan, T.P., Kemshead, J.T., Doherty, D., and F.S. Walsh
(1983). J. Neuroimmunology 5, 111-123.
Fontana, A., Hengartner, H., de Tribolet, N., and E. Weber, (1984-1). J.
Immunology, 132, 1837-1844.
Fontana, A., Fierz, W., and H. Wekerle (1984-2). Nature 307, 273-276.
Gately, M.K., Glaser, M., Dick, S.J., Meitetal, R.W., and P.L. Kornblith
(1982). J.N.C.I., 69, 1245-1254.
Gerosa, M., Chilosi, M., Iannucci, A., Montagna, M., Andrighetto,
G.C.,Stevanoni, G., and G. Tridente (1984). J. Neurooncology, 2, 451-461.
Kemshead, J.T., Ritter, M.A., Cotmore, S.F., and M.F. Greaves (1982). Brain
Research 236, 451-461.
Kennet, R.H. and F.M. Gilbert (1978). Science 203, 1120-1121.
Köhler, G., and C. Milstein (1975). Nature, 256, 495-497.
Mahaley, M.S. (1972). Prog. Exp. Tumor Res., 17, 31-39.
Martin-Achard, A., Diserens, A.C., de Tribolet, N., and S. Carrel (1980).
Int. J. Cancer, 25, 219-224.
Neuwelt, E.A. (1984). Prog. Exp. Tumor Res. 28, 51-66.
Pfreundschuh, M., Shiku, H., Takahashi, T., Ransohoff, J., Ottgen, H.F., and
Old, L. (1978). Proc. Natl. Acad. Sci. USA, 75, 5122-5126.
Piguet, V., Diserens, A.C., Carrel, S., Mach, J.P., and N. de Tribolet (1985).
Springer Seminars in Immunopathology, 8, 111-127.
Rapoport, S.I., Blood Brain Barrier in Physiology and Medicine. Raven Press,
New York, 1976.
Schnegg, J.F., de Tribolet, N., Diserens, A.C., Martin-Achard, A., and S.
Carrel (1981). Int. J. Cancer, 28, 265-269.
Schreyer, M., Hamou, M.F., Carrel, S., Mach, J.P., and N. de Tribolet (1985).
Markers of Human Neuroectodermal Tumors, CRC Press, Boca Raton, in press.
Seeger, R.C., Rosenblatt, H.M., Imai, S.A., and S. Ferrone (1981). Cancer
Res., 41, 2712-2717.
Seeger, R.C., Damon, Y.L., Rayner, S.A., and F. Hoover (1982). J.
Immunology, 128, 983-989.
Shapiro, J.R., Yung, W.A., and W.R. Shapiro (1981). Cancer Res., 41, 23-59.
Unanue, E.R., Beller, D.I., Lu, C.Y., and P.M. Allen (1984). J. of
Immunology, 132, 1-14.
Wikstrand, C.J., Bigner, S.H., and D.D. Bigner (1983). Cancer Res., 43,
3327-3340.
Wikstrand, C.J., Mahley, M.S., and D.D. Bigner (1977). Cancer Res., 37,
4267-4275.
Yamasaki, T., Yamasaki, J., Wanda, H., Watanabe, Y., Namba, Y., and M. Hanadka
(1984). Cancer Res., 44, 1776-1783.

Toward Medulloblastoma Cell Lines: Preliminary Report

M. A. Gerosa*, M. L. Rosenblum**,
G. Stevanoni***, M. Tommasi***,
E. Raimondi****, A. Nicolato*, A. Bricolo* and
G. Tridente***

*Department of Neurosurgery, University of Verona, Verona, Italy
**Brain Tumor Research Center, University of California San
Francisco, San Francisco, USA
***Department of Immunology, University of Verona,
Verona, Italy
****Department of Genetics, University of Pavia, Pavia, Italy

ABSTRACT

Medulloblastomas hardly grow in vitro. To date, only in a few cases have long-term cultures of this tumor been obtained. A medulloblastoma (MB) research program, designed with the aim of developing MB cell lines is presented. During the first 10 months of the project, 9 primary and 2 recurrent cerebellar MBs have been cultured in vitro; only in 3 cases has prolonged subculturing been successful, one of the 'putative' cell lines presently being in p12 (PF 161) and the others in p7 (OP 187) and p6 (CB 193) respectively. In all cases a considerable pleomorphism has been observed during in vitro growth.

The preliminary results of phenotypic characterization by immunohistochemical techniques indicate poorly differentiated cell populations, highly positive for Vimentin staining, with smaller fractions of cells positive for neurofilaments, neuron-specific enolase and GFAP staining. After genotypic characterization of the 'older' culture (PF 161) no markers of gene amplification have been observed. Chromosome counts have shown a bi-modal peak distribution with a high incidence of endoreduplications (11%).

KEYWORDS

Medulloblastoma; cell culture; clonogenic assay; immunohistochemistry; GFAP; GE_2; Vimentin; neurofilaments; neuron-specific enolase; HLA-DR; gene amplification; endoreduplication.

INTRODUCTION

Medulloblastoma (MB) is a highly malignant brain tumor currently accounting for 15-30% of all pediatric C.N.S. malignancies (Farwell et al, 1977; Russell and Rubinstein, 1977; Choux et al, 1982).

The histogenesis and the differentiating capabilities of this cerebellar neoplasm have been extensively discussed, with some authors endorsing the theory of an altogether poorly differentiated neuro-epithelial tumor (Elvidge et al, 1937; Rubinstein and Northfield, 1964; Scharenberg and Liss, 1969; Bailey, 1971; Rubinstein, 1972), and others suggesting a possible mesenchymal origin (Gullotta, 1967; Kersting, 1968; Matakas et al, 1970; Gullotta and Kersting, 1972).

It is generally accepted that the lack of well characterized in vitro models has consistently hampered major advances both in biological investigations and in devising innovative treatments (McAllister et al, 1977; Weichselbaum et al, 1977; Zeltzer et al, 1984).

To date, despite several repeated attempts, only a small number of MB cultures have survived for prolonged periods (Manuelidis, 1965; Barker et al, 1972), and only one established cell line has been obtained from explanted human MB, i.E. the TE 671 line obtained by McAllister et al (McAllister et al, 1977). The reasons for this failure are not clear.

Our current MB project at Verona University has been designed in order to develop permanent human MB cell lines, to characterize their genotypes and phenotypes, to clone a fraction of their cell population, and eventually to produce anti-MB monoclonal antibodies.

The preliminary results with presently growing short- and long-term cultures of MB explants are reported.

MATERIALS AND METHODS

The main steps of our MB project are summarized in Table 1. Some of these topics deserve specific comment.

Table 1. MB project: planned investigations.

A. In vitro growth
         - monolayer
         - agar

B. In vitro chemosensitivity testing

C. Phenotypic characterization
         - immunohistochemistry
         - ultrastructure
         - biochemistry

D. Genotypic characteriziation
         - karyotype
         - banding

E. Tumorigenicity studies (nude mice)

F. Production of anti-MB monoclonal antibodies

A. Monolayer cultures

The procedure for obtaining human brain tumor cultures from surgical specimens according to the 'Human Brain Tumor Stem Cell Assay" (HBTSCA) has been reported in detail (Rosenblum et al, 1976; Rosenblum et al, 1978; Rosenblum et al, 1983). Briefly, tumor biopsies are minced within 3 hours into pieces of less than 1 cu.mm, which are subsequently disaggregated into a single cell suspension with a 30 min. exposure at 37°C to an enzyme cocktail (pronase 0.05% PKU/mg; collagenase 0.02% of 125 U/mg; DNAse 0.02% of $7x10^4$ dornase units/mg). After filtration to remove nondigested particles, the single cell suspension is divided into 25/75 cm^2 tissue culture flasks, and cells are incubated at 37°C in a humidified atmosphere with 5% CO_2 in an enriched medium containing Eagle's Minimum Essential Medium (MEM), nonessential amino acids, glutamine, gentamycin 0.5%, and 20% Fetal Calf Serum.

For routine culture establishment, flasks are incubated as long as required to obtain healthy monolayer cell growth with medium changes as necessary; by that time the monolayer is treated with a disaggregating solution (trypsin 0.25% + EDTA 1.5 mg/ml), the saturation density (SD) is calculated, and the cell suspensions are either frozen in liquid nitrogen or processed for subculturing with a split ratio of 1:2-1:4.

For cell survival studies and for analysis of the 'Colony Forming Efficiency' (CFE), heavily X-irradiated (4,000 Rads) 9L-gliosarcoma 'feeder' cells are added to tumor cells in 5 cm Petri dishes ($5x10^4$/dish), which are incubated for 2-4 weeks without changing the medium (Rosenblum et al, 1976; Rosenblum et al, 1978; Rosenblum et al, 1983). Colonies (distinct groups of more than 25 cells with similar morphology) develop from single cells that have retained the capacity for in vitro proliferation. Using the same assay, plating efficiency (PE) on solid substrate is determined by counting colonies of 5 or more cells 14 days after plating $5x10^2$ and $5x10^3$ cells.

B. Agar cultures

The basic aim of culturing MB explants in soft agar is to compare the in vitro growth and PE of this tumor in a monolayer system with the corresponding parameters obtained in a semisolid medium inhibiting fibroblast proliferation. Several agar suspension culture techniques have been described in the past (McPherson, 1964; Salmon, 1980; Dendy and Hill, 1984). For the purposes of this investigation the 'replenishable soft agar colony assay' (Courtenay, 1984) has been adopted with minor modifications. In selected cases, the results obtained with this system will be compared with those provided by the Hamburger-Salmon technique (Salmon, 1980), i.e. using agar 0.5% in the bottom layer and 0.3% in the upper layer.

C. In vitro chemosensitivity testing

In vitro chemosensitivity studies are performed on early (1-4) and late (over 5) culture passages according to HBTSCA (Rosenblum et al, 1976; Rosenblum et al, 1978; Rosenblum et al, 1983; Rosenblum et al, 1984), using a panel of antitumor agents including 1,3 bis(2-chloroethyl)-1-nitrosourea (BCNU), cis-diammine-dichloro-platinum(II) (CDDP), beta and gamma interferon. Briefly, exponentially growing cell cultures are exposed to various concentrations of BCNU, CDDP or platinum analogues (i.e. drugs with a half-life shorter than 1 hour (Schein et al, 1978; Prestayko et al, 1980) for 2 hours at 37°C. Cell cultures are then washed and trypsinized, and differential cell concentrations are seeded in 60 mm Petri dishes with the complete medium described above, and a 'feeder' layer of heavily irradiated 9L-gliosarcoma cells. The CFE of the tumor is determined after an incubation of 2-4 weeks at 37°C in a 95% air/5% CO_2 atmosphere (Rosenblum et al, 1976; Rosenblum et al, 1978; Rosenblum et al, 1983).

A partially different procedure is used for in vitro treatment with beta and gamma interferon, the half-life of these two drugs being much longer (23-30 hr) (Baron et al, 1982; Cook et al, 1983). Graded concentrations of these agents are administered to exponentially growing MB cultures according to a schedule of continuous treatment.

To evaluate in vitro cytotoxicity, three to four replicate dishes are analyzed for each drug dose; untreated control dishes are similarly prepared. The ratio between the CFEs of treated and untreated cells is recorded as the surviving fraction of clonogenic cells at each drug dose; the surviving fraction is plotted against drug concentrations for analysis of the dose response (Rosenblum et al, 1976; Rosenblum et al, 1978; Rosenblum et al, 1983).

D. Phenotypic characterization of cells and colonies

- Immunohistochemistry

The panel of immunohistochemical markers investigated and the positivity scores are summarized in Table 2.

Table 2. Immunohistochemical markers.

A. Panel

Glial fibrillary acidic protein (GFAP)
Vimentin (VM)
Neurofilaments (NF)
Neuron-specific enolase (NSE)
Antiglioma monoclonal antibody: GE_2 (ref. 43)
Human HLA.ABC
        HLA.DR

B. Score

−   No positive cells
(+) $< 1\%$
+   1-10%
++   10-50%
+++ $> 50\%$

The basic procedure for routine (every 5-6 passages) characterization of cultures and colonies are essentially similar for all these markers and have been reported in detail (Tubbs et al, 1981; Bonnin and Rubinstein, 1984). For the purposes of this study, the culture passage to be examined is trypsinized and a fraction of the single cell suspension is plated into chamber slides (approximately 70,000 cells/chamber with 1.5 ml of complete medium) and incubated as usual (37°C; 5% CO_2) for 2-4 days. When the cells are close to confluence, the culture medium is removed, the slides are carefully washed with Phosphate Buffer Saline (PBS) and fixed in a chloroform/acetone 1:1 mixture for 10 min. After fixation the slides are air-dried and frozen at -20°C. Before the staining procedure, a post-fixation is performed: slides are fixed in PLP (para-formaldehyde-lysine-sodium periodate) for 10 min., washed in PBS and covered in a moist chamber with 100 μl of diluted normal human serum in order to prevent unpecific binding of immunoglobulins to Fc receptors. After a 15 min. incubation at room temperature, the normal human serum is removed and the slides are incubated with the primary antibody (mostly mouse monoclonal antibodies). An hour later, the slides are incubated again for 30 min. with a horseradish-peroxidase-conjugated 'second layer' (mostly rabbit antimouse immunoglobulin antibody).

The final peroxidase staining is performed using a mixture of 3'-3 diammino-benzidine dissolved in ethylene glycol monoethyl ether and H_2O_2. In all cases the slides are counterstained with hematoxylin.

- Other techniques

Conventional routine techniques are used to investigate the pathology and the ultrastructural aspects of these cultures.

Owing to the well-known radiosensitivity of medulloblastomas, our biochemical studies are mainly focused on the analysis of the free-radical scavenger enzymes in these cultured cells. The panel of enzymes currently under investigation includes superoxide dismutase, catalase, glutathion reductase and glutathion peroxidase (Rosenblum et al, 1984).

E. Genotypic characterization

Chromosome count and karyotyping are regularly performed (every 5-6 passages) directly on log-phase monolayer cultures. Cells are grown on cover slips in Minimum Essential Medium supplemented with 20% fetal calf serum, streptomycin (100 mg/ml) and penicillin (100 I.U./ml). When confluent cells cover approximately 50% of the slide surface and a large numebr of mitoses are shown at microscopic observation, Colcemid (Gibco Lab., Grand Island Biological Co.) is added at a final concentration of 0.3 ug/ml for 3 hours. Subsequently the cell culture is treated with 0.7% sodium citrate hypotonic solution for 15 min and then fixed using a standard 3:1 methanol/acetic acid preparation directly on adherent cells. Slides are either stained with Giemsa or G-banded (Seabright, 1972). Modal chromosome numbers are determined on samples of at least 30 metaphases.

Adequately spread and G-banded modal metaphases are photographed and karyotyped.

F. Tumorigenicity studies

The main techniques for tumorigenicity testing in nude mice have been described (Giovanella et al, 1974; Bigner et al, 1981).

In our protocol, tumor cell suspensions obtained from putatively developing MB cell lines, over p15, will be injected into the animal. Mice will be routinely sacrificed when tumors are formed, and the tumor mass will be removed aseptically for cell culture, phenotypic and genotypic characterization.

The final goals of this project remain the production of anti-MB monoclonal antibodies, and the cloning of these highly heterogeneous tumor cell populations.

PRELIMINARY RESULTS

During the first year of this research program, 9 primary and 2 recurrent cerebellar medulloblastomas have been cultured in vitro. So far, only in 3 cases of primary MB (PF 161,OP 187, CB 193) has prolonged subculturing been successful. PF 161, the 'leader', presently at p12, is putatively becoming an MB cell line, whereas OP 187 and CB 193 are still at an earlier culture stage (p7 and p6 respectively).

In all these cases histology confirmed a 'classic' medulloblastoma with no desmoplastic aspects, as shown in Table 3. Morphological observation of cultured cells invariably showed a pleomorphic cell population (Figs. 1-2) with at least 3-4 major phenotypes: rounded, spindle-shaped, bi-tripolar large undifferentiated cells (the most frequent, with unusually low saturation densities).

Table 3. Basic phenotypes of the 3 subcultures.

	Morphology in vitro	Saturation Density (cells/cm^2)	Plating Efficiency (%)
PF 161	Pleomorphic: - Rounded - Spindle-shaped - Large bi-tripolar - Giant	p7 (5.4×10^4)	p7 (0.8)
OP 187	"	p4 (6.2×10^4)	-
CB 193	"	p4 (8.3×10^4)	-

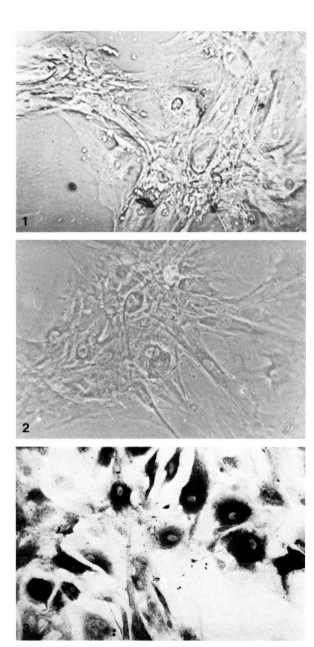

Figs. 1–2. *In vitro* growth of PF 161 p2 (Fig. 1) and OP 187 p3 (Fig. 2): pleomorphism of the cell population. (× 400).

Fig. 3. PF 161 p3 — GE$_2$ staining.
Several cells, mostly large and rounded, show an intense GE$_2$ positivity.

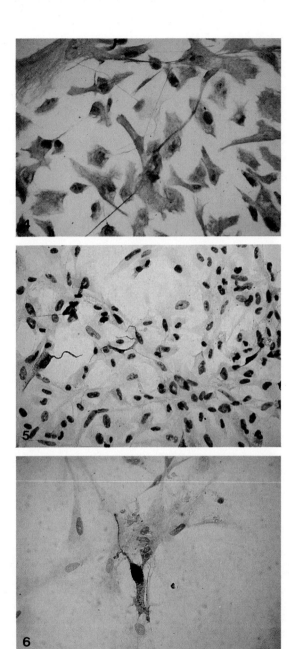

Fig. 4. PF 161 p7 — VM staining.
Pronounced morphological heterogeneity. A large majority of cells, however, are Vimentin-positive.

Fig. 5. CB 193 pl — GFAP staining.
A fraction of GFAP-positive, mature, astrocyte-like elements, surrounded by proliferating neoplastic cells.

Fig. 6. OP 187 p2 — HLA-DR staining.
One isolated DR+ cell.

Preliminary results of the immunohistochemical characterization of these cultures are summarized in Table 4.

Table 4. Immunohistochemical markers.

	PF 161			OP 187		CB 193	
	p3	p7	p11	p2	p6	p1	p5
GFAP	++	+	−	+	−	+	+
VM	+++	+++	+++	+++	+++	+++	+++
NF	++	++	++	+	+	++	+
NSE	+	+	−	+	(+)	+	(+)
GE$_2$	++	+++	++	++	+++	+++	++
Human HLA.ABC	+++	+++	+++	+++	+++	+++	+++
HLA.DR	(+)	(+)	−	(+)	+	+	+

Some of the histochemical markers (Vimentin, GE$_2$, neurofilaments) were consistently positive in all culture passages (Figs. 3–4) of the 3 tumors tested.

In the early culture passages, an average of 1–10% of the cells was found to be positive for glial fibrillary acidic protein (GFAP) (Fig. 5); these were mostly mature, astrocytic-like elements that gradually disappeared with subculturing. A similar statistical incidence (1–5%) was shown by NSE immunostaining: a small fraction of cells bearing this isoenzyme was detectable in all 3 culture sets.

Positivity for human HLA.ABC (major histocompatibility complex) was maintained, whereas HLA.DR antigens were present in a strict minority of cells in the early passages of PF 161 and OP 193: however, DR positivity was subsequently lost (Fig. 6).

To date, results of karyological analysis are available only for PF 161 (p7). The chromosome counts show a bi-modal peak distribution (Fig. 7) with a prevalent near-diploid population and a second peak in the tetraploid population. This is at least partly explained by the high incidence (11%) of endoreduplications that has been found in these cells.

No markers of gene amplification (HSR, DMs) have been observed.

CHROMOSOME NUMBER DISTRIBUTION

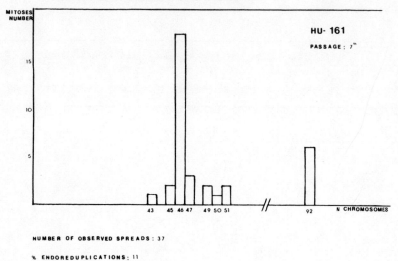

Fig. 7. PF 161 p7 - chromosome count.
Bi-modal peak distribution.

DISCUSSION

A large series of human malignant glioma cell lines has been established over the past decades (Pontén, 1975; Bigner et al, 1981; Shapiro et al, 1981), whereas only in limited cases have long-term in vitro MB cultures been obtained (Manuelidis, 1965; Barker et al, 1972; Westermark et al, 1973; Mac Allister et al, 1977) (Table 5). Several possible reasons might explain this failure.

According to Pontén (Pontén, 1975), in 1975 too few MB biopsies had been cultured. To date, some one hundred attempts have been made (Zeltzer et al, 1984), even though the size of the specimen is often too small if compared with the routine size of gliomas. Furthermore, MB cells show an 'intrinsic' diffi-culty to attach to the surface of the culture vessels as well as to proliferate in semisolid media (Westermark et al, 1973; Lumsden, 1974; Pontén, 1975).

Finally, it should be emphasized that MBs are usually characterized by a high degree of heterogeneity (Lumsden, 1974; Rubinstein, 1974; Russell and Rubin-stein, 1977; Camins et al, 1980; Zeltzer et al, 1984) and by a remarkable potential for differentiation along neuro-glial (Rubinstein, 1974; Camins et al, 1980; Palmer et al, 1981; Zeltzer et al, 1984), neuroblastic (Bailey, 1971; Rubinstein, 1974; Rubinstein et al, 1974; Camins et al, 1980; Palmer et al, 1981) and mesenchymal (Gullotta, 1967; Kersting, 1968; Matakas et al, 1970;

Gullotta and Kersting, 1972) cell lines. These differentiating potentialities might significantly hamper the development of tumor stem lines in vitro.

Table 5. MB long-term cultures.

Author	Number of MBs grown in vitro	Results
Manuelidis (ref. 24)	8	2 growing 1 surviving for 131 days
Barker (ref. 2)	6	Cont. cell cultures surviving 42-1,355 days
McAllister (ref. 22)	TE 671 : Hu MB cell line	

Our preliminary observations seem to confirm the gross phenotypic heterogeneity of this tumour, with pronounced cellular pleomorphism, which should be more typical of glial than of neuronal tumor cell lines (Rubinstein, 1974; Russell and Rubinstein, 1977; Palmer et al, 1981; Baron et al, 1982; Zeltzer et al, 1984). The multiplicity of cell types observed might be a consequence of PF 161, OP 187 and CB 193 being uncloned cell populations. However, recent evidence indicates that whenever TE 671, i.e. the only MB cell line available to date, was mechanically cloned, the resulting progeny consisted of all 6 cell phenotypes observed in the continuous culture (Zeltzer et al, 1984), thereby suggesting that, despite the multiple phenotypic variants, the transformation event in MB cell lines might essentially affect a single oncotype (Zeltzer et al, 1984).

Results of immunohistochemical studies appear to indicate that the majority of cells in all 3 of these putative MB lines are poorly differentiated anaplastic elements. Vimentin staining is highly positive in a large percentage of cells, and positivity is maintained during subculturing. Cells are mostly positive for GE_2: this might be explained by the presence of tumor-associated antigens cross-reacting with gliomas, by a neuro-glial differentiation of a fraction of this MB progeny (Rubinstein et al, 1974), and finally by a proliferation of pre-existing 'stromal' glial elements (Rubinstein et al, 1974). However, these latter hypotheses seem unlikely, particularly if we consider that GFAP positivity gradually disappears in these cells.

The consistent positivity for neurofilaments (NF) observed in all our studies might represent a major problem for the future of these long-term MB cultures;

indeed, the presence of NF in the cell processes and perikarya has generally been interpreted not only as a phenomenon of structural adaptation of neuroglial cells to the in vitro environment (Weinstein and Kornblith, 1971; Lumsden, 1974; Rubinstein et al, 1974; Russell and Rubinstein, 1977), but primarily as indicative of active protein synthesis in differentiating elements (Peters et al, 1970; Rubinstein et al, 1974; Velasco et al, 1985).

Neuron-specific enolase (NSE) is generally considered as a specific marker for neuronal cells (Marangos et al, 1979), this isoenzyme being currently expressed by malignant neuroblastoma cells and never by glial cytotypes (Marangos et al, 1979; Zeltzer et al, 1984). A few clusters of cells were positive for NSE in the early passages of our cultures; this might further confirm the low to barely detectable levels of the enzyme found in TE 671 using a radio-immuno-assay technique (Zeltzer et al, 1984).

A strict minority of cells bearing HLA-DR antigens was detected. However, DR+ phenotypes progressively disappeared with increasing culture passages, and their incidence in the total cell population was comparatively lower than in malignant gliomas (Gerosa et al, 1984). The potential role of these 'activated' astrocytes, possibly behaving as antigen-presenting cells, is under discussion (De Tribolet et al, 1984).

As regards the genotypic characterization of PF 161, although the reults are too preliminary to allow us to draw any conclusions, it should be noted that even this putative MB cell line shows a near-diploid chromosome number, as in the case of TE 671 (McAllister et al, 1977) and an unusually elevated rate of endoreduplications, the latter being a mitotic abnormality reportedly associated with a pronounced metastatic potential (Larizza and Schirrmarcher, 1984).

ACKNOWLEDGEMENTS

This research was supported in part by grants from the Italian National Research Council (C.N.R.), Rome, under the Oncological Research Project, and from the Regione Veneto, Venice, Italy. The authors wish to express their gratitude to Dr. Stephan Carrel of the Ludwig Institute for Cancer Research, Lausanne, for kindly providing the GE_2 monoclonal antibody, to Mrs. Liliana Pascoli for her technical assistance, and to Mr. Anthony Steele for editing the text of this paper.

REFERENCES

1. Bailey O.T. (1971). In 'Pathology of the Nervous System', J. Minckler ed., vol. 2, pp.2071-2081, Mac Graw-Hill, New York, N.Y.
2. Barker M., Wilson C.B., Hoshino T. (1972). In 'The Experimental Biology of Brain Tumors', W.M. Kirsch, E.G. Paoletti and P. Paoletti eds., pp.57-84, Charles C. Thomas Publ., Springfield, Ill.
3. Baron S., Dianzani F., Stanton G.J. (1982). Texas Rep. Biol. Med. 41, Part 1.
4. Biedler J.L., Helson L., Spengler B.A. (1973). Cancer Res. 22:2643-2652.
5. Bigner S.H., Bullard D.E., Pegram C.N., Wikstrand C.J., Bigner D.D.(1981). J. Neuropathol. Exp. Neurol. 40: 390-409.
6. Bonnin J.M., Rubinstein L.J. (1984). J. Neurosurg. 60:1121-1133.
7. Camins J.M.B., Cravioto H.M., Epstein F., Ransohoff J. (1980). Neurosurgery 6 : 398-411.
8. Choux M., Lena G. (1982). Neurochirurgie 28, Suppl. 1.
9. Cook A.W., Carter W.A., Nidzgorski F., Akhtar L.(1983). Science 219:881-883.
10. Courtenay V.D. (1984). In 'Predictive Drug Testing on Human Tumor Cells', V. Hofmann, M.E. Berens, G. Martz eds., pp. 17-35, Springer Verlag, Berlin.
11. Dendy P.P., Hill B.T. (1984). Human Tumor Drug Sensitivity Testing In Vitro: Techniques and Clinical Applications. Academic Press, New York, N.Y.
12. De Tribolet N., Piguet V., Diserens A.C., Mach J.P., Carrel S. (1984). In 'Developmental Neuroscience: Physiological, Pharmacological and Clinical Aspects', F. Caciagli, E. Giacobini and R. Paoletti eds., pp.273-279, Elsevier, Amsterdam.
13. Elvidge A.R., Penfield W., Cone W. (1937). Assoc. Res. Nerv. Dis. Proc. 16: 107-181.
14. Farwell J.R., Dohrmann G. J., Flannery J.T. (1977). Cancer 40: 3123-3132.
15. Gerosa M.A., Chilosi M., Jannucci A., Montagna M., Andrighetto G.C., Stevanoni G., Tridente G. (1984). J. Neuro-Oncol. 2: 272-273.
16. Giovannella B.C., Stehlin J.S., Williams L.J. (1974). J. Natl. Cancer Inst. 52 : 921-930.
17. Gullotta F. (1967). Acta Neuropathol. (Berlin) 8: 76-83.
18. Gullotta F., Kersting G. (1972). Virchows Arch. 356: 111-118.
19. Kersting G. (1968). In 'Progress in Neurological Surgery', H. Krayenbühl, P.E. Maspes and W.H. Sweet eds., vol. 2, pp. 165-202, Yearbook Medical Publishers, Chicago, Ill.
20. Larizza L., Schirrmarcher V. (1984). Cancer Met. Rev. 3: 193-202.
21. Lumsden C.D. (1974). In 'Handbook of Clinical Neurology', P.J. Vinken and G.W. Bruyn eds., pp. 42-103, North Holland Publ. Co., Amsterdam.
22. Mac Allister R.M., Isaacs H., Rongey R., Peer M., Au W., Soukup S.W., Gardner M.B. (1977). Int. J. Cancer 20: 206-212.
23. Mac Pherson I., Montagnier L. (1964). Virology 23: 291-294.
24. Manuelidis E.E. (1965). J. Neurosurg. 22: 368-373.
25. Marangos P.J., Schmechel D.E., Parma A., Clark R.I., Goodwin F.K. (1979). J. Neurochem. 33: 319-329.
26. Matakas F., Cervòs Navarro J., Gullotta F. (1970). Acta Neuropathol. (Berlin) 16: 271-284.
27. Palmer J.O., Kasselberg A.G., Netski M.G. (1981). J. Neurosurg. 55:161-169.
28. Peters A., Palay S.L., Webster H. de F. (1970). The fine structure of the Nervous System. The cells and their processes. Harper and Row, New York, N.Y.

29. Pontén J. (1975). In J. Fogh (ed.) 'Tumor Cells In Vitro', pp. 175-206, Plenum Press, New York-London.
30. Prestayko A.W., Crooke S.T., Carter S.K. (1980). Cisplatin: current status and new developments. Academic Press, New York.
31. Rosenblum M.L., Gerosa M.A., Bodell W.J., Talcott R.L. (1984). Progr. Exp. Tumor Res. 27: 191-214.
32. Rosenblum M.L., Gerosa M.A., Wilson C.B., Barger G.R., Pertuiset B.F., De Tribolet N., Dougherty D.V. (1983). J. Neurosurg. 58:170-176.
33. Rosenblum M.L., Knebel K.T., Vasquez D.A., Wilson C.B. (1976). Cancer Res. 36 : 3718-3725.
34. Rosenblum M.L., Vasquez D.A., Hoshino T., Wilson C.B. (1978). Cancer 41: 2305-2314.
35. Rubinstein L.J. (1972). Tumors of the Central Nervous System. Atlas of Tumor Pathology, 2nd series, Fasc. 6, pp. 130-153, Armed Forces Institute of Pathology, Washington D.C.
36. Rubinstein L.J. (1974). In P.J. Vinken & G.W. Bruyn (eds.)'Handbook of Clinical Neurology' pp. 167-193, North Holland Publ. Co. , Amsterdam.
37. Rubinstein L.J., Herman M.M., Hanbery J. W. (1974). Cancer 33: 675-690.
38. Rubinstein L.J., Northfield D.W.C. (1964). Brain 87 : 379-412.
39. Russell D.S., Rubinstein L.J. (1977). Pathology of Tumours of the Central Nervous System. 4th ed. Edward Arnold, London.
40. Salmon S.E. (1980). Cloning of Human Tumor Stem Cells. Alan R. Liss Publ., New York, N.Y.
41. Scharenberg K., Liss I. (1969). Neurectodermal Tumors of the Central and Peripheral Nervous System. Williams and Wilkins, Baltimore.
42. Schein P.S., Heal J., Green D., Wooley P.V. (1978). Antibiot. Chemother. 23: 64-75.
43. Schnegg J.F., Diserens A.C., Carrel S., Accolla R.S., De Tribolet N. (1981). Cancer Res. 41: 1209-1213.
44. Seabright M. (1972). Chromosoma (Berlin) 36: 204-210, 1972.
45. Shapiro J.R., Yung W.A., Shapiro W.R. (1981). Cancer Res. 41:2349-2359.
46. Tubbs R.R., Sheibani K., Deodhar S.D., Hawk W.A. (1981). Cleveland Clinic Quarterly 48 : 245-281.
47. Velasco M.E., Ghobrial M.W., Ross E.R. (1985). Surg. Neurol. 23: 177-182.
48. Weichselbaum R.R., Liszczak T.M., Phillips J.P., Little J.B., Epstein J., Kornblith P.L. (1977). Cancer 40: 1087-1096.
49. Weinstein R.S., Kornblith P.I. (1971). Cancer 27: 1174-1181.
50. Westermark B., Pontén J., Hugosson R. (1973). Acta Path. Microbiol. Scand. 81 : 791-805.
51. Zeltzer P.M., Schneider S.L., Von Hoff D.D. (1984). J. Neuro-Oncol. 2:35-45.

Human Brain Tumor Clonogenic Cell Assay

M. L. Rosenblum, D. V. Dougherty,
S. M. Oredsson, L. J. Martin, J. T. Rutka,
D. A. Emma and M. A. Gerosa

Brain Tumor Research Center, Department of Neurosurgery,
University of California, San Francisco USA

It is presumed that a better understanding of tumor growth and response to treatment will result from an analysis of the clonogenic cell and its survival following therapeutic manipulations.

Over the past 12 years we have been involved with the development of a human brain tumor clonogenic cell assay. The correlation of in vitro chemosensitivity trials with in vivo tumor response to nitrosoureas has suggested that we are culturing a relevant tumor cell population.

Optimal utilization of such studies should take into consideration factors such as: drug pharmacology (including the possibility of blood–brain–traverse), mechanism(s) of drug activity, drug–drug interactions and the therapeutic index.

We will present results of our tumor studies with 1,3-bis(2-chloro-ethyl)-1-nitrosourea (BCNU) and difluoro-methylornithine (DFMO) to illustrate the potential utility of the assay.

The effect of polyamine depletionby DFMO on cell proliferation and on the cytotoxicity of BCNU was studied in three human glioblastomas grown in monolayer culture (1). DFMO (generously provided by the Merrell–Dow Research Center, Cincinnati, Ohio) is an enzyme-activated irreversible inhibitor of ornithine decarboxylase that has shown the ability to potentiate BCNU cytotoxicity in BCNU-sensitive (2) but not BCNU-resistant 9L rat brain tumor cells (3). Two of the human tumors were sensitive to BCNU in vitro, while one was not. Ten and 20 mM DFMO effectively inhibited the growth of cells from all three tumors. Putrescine and spermidine were depleted to non-detectable levels while spermine was slightly elevated or paralleled control levels in all three tumors.

A colony forming efficiency assay (4) was used to study the effect of polyamine depletion by 10 or 20 mM DFMO on the cytotoxicity of BCNU. Although polyamines were depleted to the same extent, BCNU cyto-toxicity was affected differently in the three glioblastomas. Polyamine

depletion by DFMO significantly increased the cytotoxicity of BCNU in the
cells from the two tumors that were sensitive to the drug. In one of these
the dose-enhancement ratio averaged 1.4 for either 10 or 20 mM DFMO
pretreatment.
In the other sensitive tumor, DFMO exerted a dose-dependent potentiation
of BCNU cytotoxicity. The dose-enhancement ratios for 10 and 20 mM DFMO
averaged 1.2 and 1.9 respectively. The increased log cell kill observed
at clinically achievable BCNU doses was directly related to the inherent
BCNU sensitivity of cells from both tumors.

Furthermore, DFMO decreased the shoulder of the BCNU dose-response
curves of both sensitive tumors. In contrast, polyamine depletion did not
affect the cytotoxicity of BCNU for cells from the BCNU-resistant glioblastoma.

Previous comparisons of in vitro clonogenic cell survival and in situ
tumor response to BCNU (4) have suggested that approximately half of all
brain tumors harbor predominantly BCNU-sensitive and half predominantly
BCNU-resistant cells. Half of the tumors with BCNU-sensitive cells (one-
quarter of the total cases) did not demonstrate a clinical response to BCNU,
whereas the other half responded. Therefore, since DFMO pretreatment
appears to potentiate only BCNU-sensitive cells, we would predict an additional response rate of approximately 25% (those cases with sensitive cells that
would not respond to BCNU when given alone). This assumption is, of course,
extremely speculative and depends upon the influence of many factors
present in situ that have not been taken into account with the in vitro
studies. Nevertheless, the observations offer a preclinical estimate of
treatment efficacy which, if corroborated by future clinical studies, would
provide an impetus for similar investigations in the future.

The growth of a patient's tumor and its response to treatment modalities will depend upon several factors that are specific to the environment
within the solid neoplasm. The local environment will be influenced by
blood flow which might vary from region to region and result in differences
including: tissue oxygenation and pH, the concentration of nutrients and
endocrine-like growth factors, and in the removal of the toxic by-products
of cell division and lysis. The growth and differentiation of a tumor cell
might be modified by associations with other tumor- and non-tumor cells
and with the extracellular matrix. Finally, tumor growth in situ is a
composite of the actual proliferation of cells based upon their inherent
kinetic potential and cell loss due both to ischemia and the host's immune
system. We would suggest that some of the poor correlations noted between
culture evaluation of chemosensitivity and patient response occurs as a
consequence of the markedly different in vitro and in vivo environments.
We are convinced that studies of clonogenic cell survival will eventually
play a major role in selecting new, effective chemotherapeutic agents for
the treatment of malignant brain tumors.
The studies with BCNU and DFMO as described here are examples of the
types of preclinical evaluations that are possible using the clonogenic cell
assay for human brain tumors. This goal should be positively influenced
by optimization of tumor growth and treatment conditions, by more realistic
pharmacokinetic considerations and by concurrent studies of normal tissue
toxicity.

REFERENCES

1. Rosenblum M.L., Vasquez D.A., Hoshino T., Wilson C.B. (1978).
   Cancer 41: 2305-2314.
2. Hung D.T., Deen D.F., Seidenfeld J., Marton L.J. (1981).
   Cancer Res. 41: 2783-2785.
3. Oredsson S.M., Tofilon P.J., Feuerstein B.J., Deen D.F., Rosenblum M.,
   Marton L.J. (1983). Cancer Res. 43: 3576-3578.
4. Rosenblum M.L., Gerosa M.A., Wilson C.B., Barger G.R., Pertuiset B.F.
   De Tribolet N., Dougherty D.V. (1983). J. Neurosurg. 58: 170-176.

In Vitro Chemosensitivity Testing of Human Brain Tumours Using Multicellular Spheroids

J. L. Darling, N. Oktar and D. G. T. Thomas

Gough-Cooper Department of Neurological Surgery, Institute of
Neurology, National Hospital, Queen Square,
London WC1N 3BG, UK

INTRODUCTION

Although monolayer cultures of human glioma have proved to be a
most important tool for investigating the effects of cytotoxic
drugs, from the point of view of providing an accurate model for
the intact tumour, they suffer from a number of disadvantages.
From results obtained with animal models, it is clear that
inherent cellular sensitivity is only one factor which determines
response to cytotoxic agents. The structure of the tumour itself
is capable of influencing the response of cells within it. This
effect can be mediated through a number of mechanisms. The
penetration of oxygen and nutrients are non-uniform within a
tumour. Certainly, cells which lie close to capillaries receive
adequate supplies of oxygen and nutrients, although the further a
cell is from a capillary, the more likely it is to be deprived of
nutrients (Tannock, 1968). Cells far removed from a capillary may
not be dead, but simply in a resting state, from which they can
be revived if conditions become more favourable and experimental
evidence from animal studies confirms that these cells can grow
to form tumours (Goldacre, 1977). The influence of capillary
proximity presumably accounts for the large number of cells in
cerebral tumours which are not in cycle. Typically, the growth
fraction of high-grade gliomas is of the order of only 10-30%
(Hoshino et al., 1975).

Drug penetration in brain material is very poor (Levin, 1979),
perhaps only of the order of a few millimetres, even from a
leaky, well perfused tumour, if the capillary permeability of
that brain region is low, preventing the drug from crossing the
capillaries in that region. Certainly, experimental evidence
using intracerebral model systems such as the 9L gliosarcoma and
the Walker 256 carcinosarcoma indicate that the transcapillary
exchange in brain immediately adjacent to the tumour was less
than that observed in unaffected brain (Levin et al., 1975). The
mechanism for this is unclear, although this impaired penetration
may explain the relative ineffectiveness of water soluble

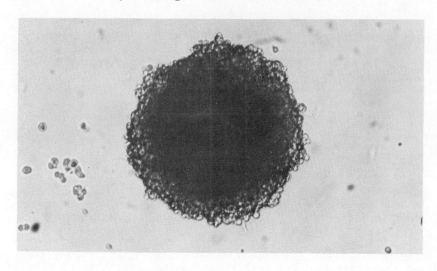

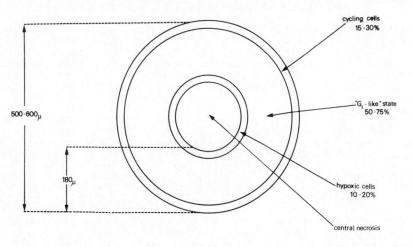

FIGURE 1.

A. A multicellular spheroid derived from the human glioma cell line U251 MG.
B. Schematic representation of a section through a typical spheroid indicating
the different regions of cell cycle activity and depicting the development
of an area of central necrosis once a critical diameter has been reached.

TABLE 1.   COMPARISON OF THREE DIMENSIONAL TUMOUR MODEL
           SYSTEMS - ORGAN CULTURE AND MULTICELLULAR SPHEROIDS

	Organ culture	Multicellular tumour spheroids
Tumour heterogeneity	Preserved although possibility of sampling error	Possibly preserved, although composition of spheroids from primary tumours unknown.
Chemosensitivity	Difficult to measure - only methods like histology, isotope uptake and metabolic activity applicable	Range of endpoints available, CFE, volume growth delay, spheroid outgrowth
Presence of normal cells	Yes, may contribute to observed chemo-therapeutic effect	Unknown
Technical aspects and cost	Complex - many technical points eg pH, tissue handling, gas phase osmolarity, substrate, temperature can influence outcome. Cost high and scale up difficult	Usually simple - requires no special equipment. Reproducible. Cost low. Scale up easy
Geometry in relation to sensitivity	Difficult to assess	Easy to assess using sequential disagg-regation techniques
Growth in vitro	Minimal	Yes
Comparison of neoplastic and normal tissue	Possible	May not be possible
Applicability to a wide range of tumour types	May be possible although growth conditions may be unique for each tumour type	May be possible (?)

cytotoxic drugs in brain tumour chemotherapy. It is important, therefore, to develop in vitro models to investigate the extracellular penetration of cytotoxic drugs.

It is also likely that within a brain tumour the extra- and intracellular microenvironment (pO_2, extracellular pH, etc.) may be different from that in normal brain and this will affect drug metabolism or stability.

Likewise, the three dimensional structure of a tumour favours the development of intercellular junctions through which cells are metabolically coupled. The ability of cells to "cooperate" in this way is responsible for the "contact effect" observed in spheroids treated with ionising radiation (Durand and Sutherland, 1972).

Spheroids provide an ideal model for the experimental investigation of some of the structural features of tumours which influence drug and radiation sensitivity (Figure 1A). There is distribution of cell cycle characteristics which is broadly in agreement with those found in tumours (Wibe et al., 1981). Multicellular spheroids adopt a morphological pattern which is similar to that observed in tumours. A thin layer of rapidly proliferating cells forming the outer shell of the spheroid, while as the distance between the surface and a cell increases, cells become arrested in a G_1-like state, then an area of truely hypoxic cells develop which, if the diameter of the spheroid begins to exceed a critical diameter, becomes a central necrotic core (Figure 1B). It is also possible to measure microenvironmental factors in indvidual spheroids using pH microelectrodes and ion-selective electrodes (Acker, 1984) as well as measuring oxygen tensions (Mueller Klieser and Sutherland, 1982). Drug penetration into spheroids can also be determined using autoradiography (West et al., 1980; Nederman et al., 1981).

Of course, there is nothing new about three dimensional cultures of human brain tumours. Organ cultures have been produced from a variety of intracranial tumours and the morphology and differentiation (Rubinstein et al., 1973; Rubinstein and Herman, 1975), cell kinetics (Hess et al., 1983) and drug sensitivity (Saez et al., 1977) have been investigated. There are, however, disadvantages associated with the use of these cultures. Table 1 details some of the advantages of spheroids over organ culture systems.

MATERIALS AND METHODS

Preparation of MTS from human tumour biopsies using liquid overlay techniques.

Tumour biopsies, collected at surgery, were minced with crossed scalpels and disaggregated with collagenase (Morgan et al., 1983; Darling et al., 1983). The resultant cell suspension was diluted to 500,000 cells/ml in growth medium (Ham's F-10, supplemented with 10% foetal calf serum, penicillin and streptomycin and buffered with 20 mM HEPES). Five millilitres of this cell suspension was intoduced into a 25 cm^2 plastic cell culture flask base-coated with 3 mls of agar (0.5% w/v Bacto or Noble agar in growth medium). After 2 - 3 days in culture, the cellular aggregates were removed from the flask and placed in a fresh agar-coated flask as there was a tendency for single cells to migrate under the agar and form a monolayer on the base of the flask. Following 7 - 10 days further incubation, when the spheroids were 100 - 200 μm in diameter, they could be distributed individually, using a fine-bore Pasteur pipette, to agar-coated wells on a 24- or 96-well microtitration plate for either drug sensitivity or growth curve studies.

Determination of drug sensitivity

Spheroids were treated in situ with appropriate concentrations of drug or drug vehicle for 24 hours and carefully washed with growth medium. For growth curve studies or growth delay determinations, spheroid size was assessed using a precalibrated eyepiece micrometer in an inverted microscope. Two measurements were made of the diameter perpendicular to each other and the mean diameter was used to determine the volume of the spheroid. The surviving fraction of drug-treated spheroids was determined by cloning a disaggregated cell suspension from a pool of ten drug treated or control spheroids in soft (0.3%) Litex agarose in a plastic cell culture tube. Tubes were tightly stoppered and incubated at 37°C for 20-30 days, after which the agarose plug was eased from the tube into a petri dish and the colonies counted with an inverted microscope.

RESULTS

Production of spheroids from human brain tumour biopsies

It was possible to produce some spheroids from most biopsies of malignant brain tumours (Table 2) although the number of spheroids produced tended to be relatively small. Overall, 83% of samples gave rise to spheroids but only 35% gave rise to the minimum number of spheroids required to carry out a chemosensitivity assay against even a single drug (>20, ten to be drug treated and ten to act as controls). A detailed analysis of spheroid formation in relation to tumour characteristics has been published (Darling et al., 1983). There did seem to be a correlation between tumour malignancy and spheroid formation. More spheroids were produced from grade IV astrocytomas, metastatic tumours and the highly malignant tumours of children like medulloblastoma. Conversely, fewer spheroids were produced from benign tumours and samples of "normal brain".

Production of spheroids from established brain tumour cell lines

The ability of a range of established cell lines derived from experimentally produced or spontaneous brain tumours in laboratory rodents and a range of established cell lines produced from human brain tumours to undergo spheroid formation has been determined using either the agar coated flask technique or a slow speed stirrer technique (MCS 104 microcarrier stirrer, Techne, Cambridge). All three cell lines derived from the spontaneous VM cell lines produced typical spheroids although two cell lines derived from nitrosourea-induced brain tumours produced small, atypical spheroids (Table 4). While all the human established cell lines produced spheroids, those produced from the medulloblastoma cell line TE 671 resembled the atypical spheroids produced from chemically-induced rodent brain tumours (Table 3). There did not seem to be a relationship between the ability to form spheroids and tumourigenicity or the expression of glial-related phenotypic markers.

TABLE 2. FORMATION OF MULTICELLULAR SPHEROIDS FROM HUMAN BRAIN TUMOURS

Tumour type	% of tumours producing spheroids			
	> 50/flask *	21-50/flask	< 20/flask	0/flask
IV astrocytomas (n=15)	20	20	47	13
III astrocytomas (n=12)	8	33	33	26
I-II astrocytomas (n=3)	0	0	66	33
metastatic tumours (n=5)**	60	20	20	0
brain tumours from children (n=5)***	40	40	20	0
benign tumours or cerebral lymphomas (n=4)**	0	0	100	0
non tumour (n=2)**	0	0	50	50

*   Spheroids/ 25 cm^2 agar-coated flask
**   See Darling et al. (1983) for details
*** Three medulloblastomas, a grade II astrocytoma and an ependymoma

TABLE 3. ESTABLISHED HUMAN CELL LINES USED IN THIS STUDY

Cell line	Source	Glial markers	Tumourigenicity*	Spheroids
U251 MG	IV Astro	GFAP**	Yes	Yes
U251 MGSp	IV Astro	GFAP	No	Yes
U118 MG	IV Astro	cAMP***	Yes	Yes
TE671	Medullo	-	Yes	Small spheroids

```
*     - tumourigenic in immune deprived or suppressed animals
**    - cultures express glial fibrillary acidic protein
***   - cells in culture respond morphologically to exogenous
        dibutryl cyclic AMP.
```

TABLE 4. ESTABLISHED RODENT CELL LINES USED IN THE STUDY

Cells	Source	Glial markers	Tumourigenic*	Spheroids
C$_6$	MNU-induced	S-100	Yes	small spheroids
A5-A15	ENU-induced	Glial filaments	Yes	small spheroids
VMDk 497	Spontaneous	GFAP, GS**	Yes	Yes
VMDk 540	Spontaneous	GFAP, GS	Yes	Yes
VMDk 560	Spontaneous	GFAP, GS	Yes	Yes

```
*  - tumourigenic in syngeneic animals
** - cultures express glutamine synthetase activity
```

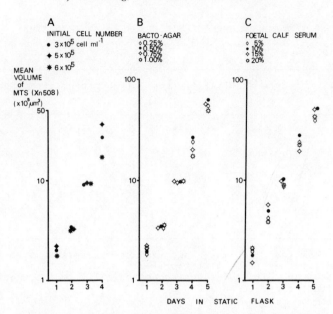

FIGURE 2.   Growth rate of spheroids derived from a xenografted human glioma
            Xn 508 initiated or maintained under different conditions.
            A. Spheroids initiated form cell suspensions of different densities.
            B. Spheroids initiated on base-coats of different agar concentrations.
            C. Spheroids grown in different foetal calf serum concentrations.

Growth of spheroids in vitro

In order to determine the influence of some environmental factors
on spheroid growth, spheroids were produced in large numbers from
a grade IV human astrocytoma which had been maintained as a
xenograft in immune-deprived mice (Xn 508, Bradley et al., 1978;
1983). It was found that neither the number of cells used to
initiate the spheroids, the concentration of agar used as the
base cover or the concentration of foetal calf serum used in the
growth medium influenced the subsequent growth rate of spheroids
(Figure 2). We have published growth curves of spheroids produced
from four human brain tumours (Darling et al., 1983) which
indicated that there was little variation in growth rate between
spheroids derived from tumours of different histology.   It was,
however, possible to show that spheroids grown in spinner flasks
did grow faster than spheroids grown in static, agar-coated
flasks. This was probably due to the enhanced oxygen or nutrient
exchange possible in stirred culture.

Chemosensitivity of MTS derived from human brain tumours

The chemosensitivity of spheroids derived from a grade IV astrocytoma were determined using growth delay as the endpoint (Figure 3). These spheroids appeared to be insensitive to procarbazine but sensitive to CCNU and markedly sensitive to vincristine. Using a clonogenic assay to determine the surviving fraction in drug treated spheroids it has been possible to demonstrate that spheroids derived from a medulloblastoma were more sensitive to VM26 than spheroids derived from a grade IV astrocytoma (Figure 4). It was also apparent that although some drugs like VM26 and L-asparaginase (L-asp) had little effect on surviving fraction in some spheroid preparations, adriamycin (ADR) appeared to be very toxic.

DISCUSSION

It has been demonstrated that it is possible to produce spheroids from a range of human brain tumour biopsies as well as from established brain tumour cell lines. Although it seems, that at present, spheroids derived directly from tumour biopsies are unlikely to be useful for individualised chemosensitivity testing because of the relatively small number produced from a small proportion of tumours. It may well be that this is due to sub-optimal culture conditions and that the addition of supplements to the culture medium might improve spheroid formation.

It is clear that it would be of considerable importance to be able to produce spheroids from a variety of histological types of human brain tumour. The use of such models may well be valuable in examining the cell biology and the therapeutic responsiveness of these tumours. In the absence of a reliable source of human tumour-derived spheroids the ability to produce large quantities from either xenografted human gliomas or from established glioma cells lines of human or rodent origin is of importance. The factors which influence the production of atypical spheroids from certain lines is unknown. Whether it is a result of chemical transformation or of culture conditions remains to be seen.

If a cell line, composed of a homogeneous population of cells, undergoes spheroid formation, cells are forced, by the constraints of three dimensional structure to adopt the characteristics of cells found in different parts of a tumour. This is therefore a powerful system for examining the effects of three dimesional structure on cell form and function. Kwok and Twentyman (1985a) using the EMT6/Ca/VJac cell line have produced spheroids which could be sequentially disaggregated into a population of cells which lay on the periphery of the spheroid and were larger and more proliferative than cells in the inner regions of the spheroid although their clonogenic potential was similar. There is, therefore, considerable adaption to position within a spheroid but once the cnstraints are removed the cells revert to their original characteristics. We do not know the composition of spheroids derived from brain tumour biopsies. Are

FIGURE 3.

An example of the chemosensitivity of spheroids measured by growth delay. Spheroids were derived from a surgical specimen of a grade IV astrocytoma

Drug exposure (24 hours)

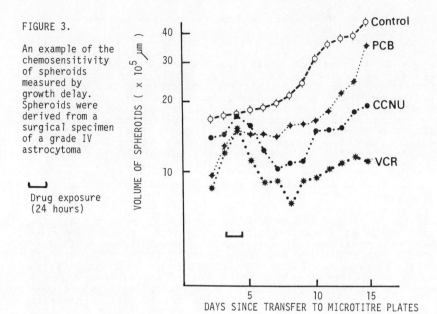

FIGURE 4.

An example of the chemosensitivity of spheroids measured by surviving fraction determination

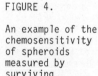

○ L-asp
▲ ADR
▼ VM26 (spheroids derived from a medulloblastoma
▽ VM26 (spheroids derived from a grade IV astrocytoma

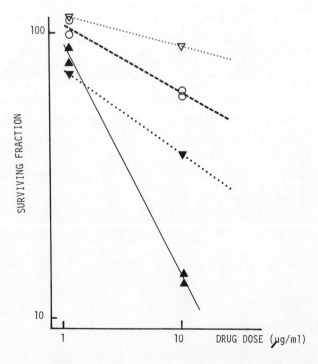

TABLE 5.   THE POTENTIAL OF MULTICELLULAR SPHEROIDS IN NEURO-
ONCOLOGY

1.   To investigate the influence of three dimensional
structure on drug resistance.

2.   To study the biology of hypoxia and develop more
effective hypoxic cell sensitisers.

3.   To investigate the role of junctional communication in
recovery from sublethal damage.

4.   Studies on three dimensional growth control.

5.   To study the effect of three dimensional structure on
cellular differentiation. Does this affect the
interaction between cell membranes and the cytoskeleton?

6.   Improve the proportion of tumour biopsies which give
rise to spheroids by manipulation of the culture
conditions. Is it possible to use these for
indvidualised chemosensitivity testing?

7.   Investigate the microenvironmental conditions within
spheroids and the influence this has on drug and
radiation sensitivity.

8.   Is drug penetration the same for a particular drug in
spheroids derived from tumours with different
histologies? Is it possible to use spheroids to screen
drugs for enhanced penetration characteristics?

9.   To investigate the relationship between cell survival
and volume growth delay in spheroids derived from
different histological types. Does this have a clinical
application?

10. Cell cycle kinetics and drug sensitivity. Investigate
the transition of resting cells to proliferating cells
and the effect of this on therapy.

all cells recruited into the spheroid or are particular cell
types (non-malignant, stromal cells) excluded from the spheroid?
Indeed, are all the spheroids produced from a single tumour
biopsy identical or is there heterogeneity between one spheroid
and the next?

Spheroids produced from any source are an interesting model
system for the study of human glioma and we have listed a number
(by no means exhaustive) of areas which warrent further
investigation using this model system (Table 5). The results
presented in this paper throw some light on the direction of
future investigations. For example, it has been reported by some
workers that adriamycin is less effective against spheroids
derived from experimentally produced rodent cell lines than when
exposed to single cells (Sutherland et al., 1979) this being
ascribed to the poor penetration of this drug into spheroids.
Factors other than penetration must account for the relative
resistance of human cervical carcinoma cell spheroids to
vincristine (Wibe, 1980) where although large quantities of drug
are able to penetrate into the spheroids, it had little cytotoxic
effect. Some of the spheroids produced from brain tumours appear
to be rather sensitive to these agents (see Figures 3 and 4).
Whether this reflects differences in drug penetration
characteristics between these spheroids or whether this is
related to the human origin or the particular histological type
of tumour from which they were derived remains to be seen. It
has been demonstrated that, for a particular drug, the response
of spheroids derived from rodent or human cell lines can be very
different (Kwok and Twentyman, 1985 a, b). We do not know what
factors are responsible for this.

The influence of three dimensional contact is unknown in
determining the chemotherapeutic responsiveness of human brain
tumours. Likewise the effect of the microenviroment within
tumours may contribute to determining drug response. Preliminary
evidence has been presented by Deen et al. (1980) suggest that
the metabolism of BCNU may be affected by the microenviromental
conditions within 9L gliosarcoma spheroids. Again, differences
between different histological types of tumour must be
investigated and correlated with the human situation.

ACKNOWLEDGEMENTS

The authors would like to thank Dr D.D. Bigner, Dr R.I. Freshney,
Dr G.J. Pilkington and Professor P.L. Lantos for supplying the
established cell lines used in this study. Dr N.J. Bradley kindly
supplied the xenografted human glioma. Financial support from
the Brain Research Trust, Cancer Research Campaign and the
British Council is gratefully acknowledged.

REFERENCES

Acker, H (1984) Rec. Results Cancer Res. **95**, 116-133.

Bradley, N.J., H.J.G. Bloom, A.J.S. Davies and S.M. Swift (1978)

Br. J. Cancer **38**, 263-272.

Bradley, N. J., J.L. Darling, N. Oktar, H.J.G. Bloom, D.G.T. Thomas and A.J.S. Davies (1983) Br. J. Cancer **48**, 819-825.

Darling, J.L., N. Oktar and D.G.T. Thomas (1983) Cell Biol. Int. Repts. **7**, 23-30.

Deen, D.F., T. Hoshino, M.E. Williams, I. Muraoka, K.D. Knebel and M. Barker (1980) J. Natn. Cancer Inst. **64**, 1373-1382.

Durand, R.E. and R.M. Sutherland (1972) Exptl. Cell Res. **71**, 75-80.

Goldacre, R.J. (1977) Br. J. Cancer **36**, 406.

Hess, J.R., J. Michaud, R.A. Sobel, M.M. Herman and L.J. Rubinstein (1983) Acta Neuropathol. (Berl.) **61**, 1-9.

Hoshino, T.M., C.B. Wilson, M.L. Rosenblum and M. Barker (1975) J. Neurosurg. **43**, 127-135.

Kwok, T.T. and P.R. Twentyman (1985a) Int. J. Cancer **35**, 675-682.

Kwok, T.T. and P.R. Twentyman (1985b) Br. J. Cancer **52** (in press).

Levin, V.A. (1979) In "Multidisciplinary Aspects of Brain Tumor Therapy", eds P. Paoletti et al. Elsevier/North Holland Biomedical Press, 165-172.

Levin, V.A., M. Freeman-Dove and H.D. Landhal (1975) Arch. Neurol. **32**, 785-791.

Morgan, D., R.I. Freshney, J.L. Darling, D.G.T. Thomas and F. Celik (1983) Br. J. Cancer **47**, 205-214.

Mueller-Klieser, W.F. and R.M. Sutherland (1982) Br. J. Cancer **45**, 256-264.

Nederman, T., J. Carlsson and M. Malmqvist (1981) In Vitro **17**, 290-298.

Rubinstein, L.J. and M.M. Herman (1975) Rec. Results Cancer Res. **51**, 35-51.

Rubinstein, L.J., M.M. Herman and V.L. Foley (1973) Am. J. Pathol. **71**, 61-80.

Saez, R.J., R.J. Campbell and E.R. Laws (1977) J. Neurosurg. **46**, 320-327.

Sutherland, R.M., H.A. Eddy, B. Bareham, K. Reich and D. Vanantwerp (1979) Int. J. Radiat. Oncol. Biol. Phys. **5**, 1225-1230.

Tannock, I.F. (1968) Br. J. Cancer **22**, 258-273.

West, G.W., R. Weichselbaum and J.B. Little (1980) Cancer Res. **40**, 3665-3668.

Wibe, E., T. Lindmo and O. Kaalhus (1981) Cell Tissue Kinet. **14**, 639-651.

Wibe, E (1980) Br. J. Cancer **42**, 937-941.

In vitro Chemosensitivity of Human Brain Tumour Tissue Cultures and Its Relationship with Relapse Free Interval

D. G. T. Thomas and J. L. Darling

Gough-Cooper Department of Neurological Surgery, Institue of
Neurology, National Hospital, Queen Square,
London WC1N 3BG, UK

INTRODUCTION

The heterogeneity of malignant gliomas has been well established.
Although this is apparent upon histological examination, more
recent analysis using modern cell biological techniques indicates
that this heterogeneity covers many aspects of cell structure and
function. Cell populations with distinct phenotypes can be
identified which differ in regard to DNA content and karyotype,
surface and cytoplasmic antigen expression and growth potential
in vitro and in vivo.

Much recent evidence has been produced to suggest that this
heterogeneity extends to sensitivity to cytotoxic drugs. In
experimental tumours there is evidence that clones of cells exist
which have different chemosensitivities (Hakansson and Trope,
1974 a,b; Barranco et al., 1978; Dexter et al., 1978; Heppner et
al., 1978) and multiple cell lines from single human neoplasms
have been shown to possess different chemosensitivities in vitro
(Barranco et al., 1972; 1973; Lotan, 1979; Dexter et al., 1981).
Studies on fresh tumour material from adenocarcinomas of the
stomach and colon (Trope et al., 1975), ovarian carcinomas
(Siracky, 1979; Trope et al., 1979) and non-Hodgkin's lymphoma
(Biorklund et al., 1980) have demonstrated that human tumours
appear to built up of clones, each of which possesses a distinct
pattern of chemosensitivity. It is, therefore, a mosaic of
clones which dictates the overall sensitivity of a tumour and is
responsible for the variation in clinical response between
patients with tumours of nominally the same histological type.

It is a general clinical observation that between 20 and 40% of
patients with malignant gliomas respond to cytotoxic drugs. It
would be of immense value to be able to predict, before
chemotherapy commences, those patients who would respond to
particular agents and those who would not. Those patients who
did not respond, at worst, would be spared the toxic effects of
chemotherapy to which they could not respond. However, using
such a test, it should be possible to identify new drug

sensitivities to enable the design of individualised chemotherapy
(Figure 1).

Although a variety of methods have been used to measure the
chemosensitivity of human glioma (Kornblith and Szypko, 1978;
Kornblith et al., 1981; Rosenblum et al., 1983) only a limited
number of clinical correlations have been reported and the impact
of these on the clinical outcome of the patients has been
difficult to assess. Using a ^{35}S-methionine uptake assay which
correlates well with monolayer cloning (Morgan et al., 1983) and
cell counting (Darling, unpublished results), we have shown that
prolonged drug treatment and recovery are necessary to produce
stable, reliable ID_{50} values. In this paper we will describe the
use of this assay to demonstrate a relationship between in vitro
chemosensitivity and clinical progress in patients with malignant
cerebral glioma.

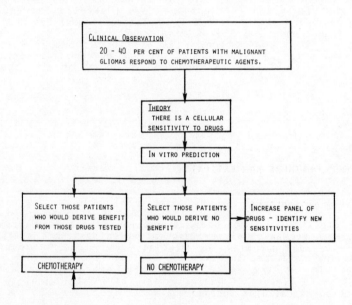

FIGURE 1.   The use of in vitro chemosensitivity assays to optimize
chemotherapy of malignant glioma.

TABLE 1. Patients with grade III and IV gliomas included in the study.

		GRADE III GLIOMAS	GRADE IV GLIOMAS	COMPARISON OF GRADE III & IV GLIOMAS
Sample size (n = 116)		51	65	-
Relapse free interval		392 days	268 days	p = 0.001*
Age at diagnosis (mean $\pm$ SD)		44.9 $\pm$ 13.4	58.3 $\pm$ 11.3	p = 0.001**
		Percentage of Groups		
Sex	Male	69	58	
	Female	31	42	NS, p = 0.3***
Tumour site	Frontal	48	32	
	Temporal	29	25	
	Parietal	23	43	NS, p = 0.07***
Operation	Partial	63	62	
	Lobectomy	37	38	NS, p = 1.0***
Radiation	0 - 4999cGy	70	78	
	5000 + cGy	30	22	NS, p = 0.47***
Steroids	Preoperative	51	55	
	Pre and postoperative	49	45	NS, p = 0.83***

* - Mantel Cox Test; ** - Students's t-test: *** - x^2 test.

MATERIALS, METHODS AND PATIENTS

Materials and methods

All materials and methods used in the collection of biopsies, initiation of monolayer cultures and the ^{35}S-methionine uptake assay have been described in detail (Thomas et al., 1979; Morgan et al., 1983).

Definition of cellular sensitivity

We have adopted a method of defining cellular sensitivity in relation to the relative sensitivity of a panel of brain tumour cultures. Over the last three years, one hunded and twenty cultures derived from malignant gliomas have been assayed for chemosensitivity against a number of drugs and this has enabled us produce "training sets" which show the range of sensitivites that can be expected for cultures derived from a particular type of tumour. The definition of in vitro sensitivity is based on

the comparison of the ID_{50} of a culture against the ID_{50}'s
produced for a panel of cultures derived from tumours of similar
histology. A culture has been defined as sensitive if it has an
ID_{50} below the median ID_{50} value for that drug of a panel of
cultures from tumours of the same histology. If the ID_{50} of a
culture lay above the median ID_{50} value for that group it was
designated as insensitive.

Patients

The characteristics and details of clinical treatment of patients
is shown in Table 1. Following radiation therapy, 116 patients
with malignant gliomas received chemotherapy, consisting of
Vincristine (VCR) 1.4 mg/m^2 as a single dose, CCNU 80 mg/m^2 as a
single dose, orally, and Procarbazine (PCB), orally, 100 mg/m^2
per day over 10 days. Patients were reviewed every six weeks and
CT scanning was performed every three months during active
therapy and every six months following its completion. Relapse
free interval (RFI) was defined as the time between operation and
deterioration. All patients included in the study had received at
least one course of chemotherapy following the completion of
radiotherapy. No attempt was made to influence therapy on the
basis of the assay result and all correlations were carried out
retrospectively.

RESULTS

Drug sensitivity in vitro: An example of a training set

As an example of a training set, the response to CCNU of 74
cultures derived from either grade III or IV gliomas is shown in
Figure 2. Routinely, 10 µg/ml was the highest concentration used
in the chemosensitivity assay. The overall range of sensitivities
was 0.027-10 µg/ml (a 370-fold range), although a majority of
cultures (39/74, 53%) had ID_{50}'s above 10 µg/ml. Of the cultures
that did have measurable ID_{50}'s, all but 6 lay in the range 1 to
10 µg/ml.

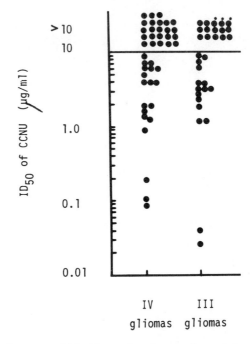

FIGURE 2.

Example of the distribution of in vitro chemo-sensitivities of a panel of 73 short-term cultures derived from grade III or IV gliomas.

* indicates a culture derived from an oligodendroglioma

IV   III

gliomas gliomas

Comparison of in vitro chemosensitivity and relapse free interval

In 40 patients it was possible to correlate in vitro data with clinical progress. The response of each culture was assessed independently to each of the drugs used clinically. The ID_{50} was compared to the appropriate training set and the culture designated a responder or non-responder as detailed above. In total 14 patients (35%) responded to CCNU, 17 (42%) responded to PCB and 16 (40%) responded to VCR. The RFI's of responders and non-responders was then compared for a particular drug using the Mantel Cox Test for the comparison of censored survival times. It was clear that the difference in RFI was significant for responders and non-responders to PCB and CCNU (p=0.02 and p=0.01 respectively) but not for VCR (p=0.5).

To further investigate the association between in vitro chemosensitvity and RFI, the entire sample was divided into three groups:

Group A   22 patients who responded to PCB and/or CCNU

Group B   18 patients who did not respond to these drugs

Group C   76 patients who had chemotherapy, but who were not tested

It was apparent that the chemosensitive group remained relapse free for longer than the non-chemosensitive group (Mantel Cox Test, p < 0.0001) and that the relapse free interval curve for group C lay between the curves of the responders and non-responders (see Thomas et al., 1985 for RFI curves). This is in agreement with the hypothesis that the untested group must be made up of in-vitro responders and non-responders although we do not know in what proportions.

It is, of course, necessary to examine the effects of patient characteristics which may act as prognostic factors as imbalances of these between groups may account for the improved RFI of the chemosensitive group. The effect of various factors in each of the groups (A, B or C) was examined as was their effect in the whole sample (A+B+C). The results are summarised in Table 2 and full details are given in Thomas et al. (1985).

TABLE 2. THE EFFECT OF PATIENT CHARACTERISTICS ON RFI

Patient characteristics which had **no** effect on RFI:

    Sex
    Side of tumour
    Extent of surgical resection
    Radiation dose
    Degree of steroid cover
    Degree of anticonvulsant cover

Patient characteristics which **did** affect RFI:

    Age   (older patients had poorer prognosis)
    Histology (grade IV tumours had poorer prognosis than
                  grade III tumours)
    Site of tumour (tumours in parietal region had poorer
                  prognosis than tumours at other sites*)

* only a prognostic sign within the **whole** sample, but not in any other sub division of the group.

It was clear that age and sex were important prognostic signs and were contributory factors in determining RFI. Site may also be of importance although its effect does not seem to be consistant. The data from groups A and B was fitted into a Cox's proportional hazard model using a forward stepwise procedure. Age, grade of tumour, site of tumour and in vitro chemosensitivity were included in the model, together with all interactions upto the third order. The model showed that even when the effects of all other factors were taken into account, chemosensitivity in vitro was still related to increased RFI.

DISCUSSION

The heterogeneity in response to cytotoxic drugs apparent between cultures derived from malignant gliomas has enabled us to identify sensitive and insensitive cultures in comparison to a training set. This is more relevant than defining sensitivity as an arbitary level of cellular inhibition at an arbitary drug concentration (Kornblith et al., 1981; Salmon et al., 1978). Often, in vivo the detailed pharmacokinetics of cytotoxic drugs are unknown and the degree of tissue penetration in the brain is only poorly understood.

Initial attempts to demonstrate a relationship between chemosensitivity in vitro and survival were undertaken by Limburg and Heckmann (1968) who showed that if the drugs predicted by the assay were used to treat patients with advanced ovarian carcinoma, survival was significantly prolonged as compared to those patients who were treated empirically. Recently, in vitro/clinical correlations have been published indicating that there is a close relationship between in vitro chemosensitivity and survival in patients with ovarian cancer using either morphological assays (Wheeler et al., 1974; Dendy 1981) or cloning assays (Alberts et al., 1984) and in patients with multiple myeloma (Durie et al., 1983). In patients with ovarian carcinoma, although there was a short-term benefit in using drugs predicted by the assay, this advantage was lost within two years (Dendy, 1981).

In the present study, it has been possible to classify patients into two groups, those who responded to PCB or CCNU in vitro and those who did not. It is also apparent that response to either of these drugs is a good prognostic sign for patients undergoing treatment with these agents. The failure of vincristine to influence RFI is surprising as this drug has shown clinical activity against some brain tumours, although it seems to be particularly effective against rapidly proliferating tumours such as medulloblastomas. Gliomas, on the other hand, have a relatively small growth fraction and it is difficult for a cell cycle specific drug to produce more than a 1 log cell kill whereas the nitrosoureas and procarbazine, agents which are active throughout the cell cycle, achieve a 3-4 log cell kill in experimental tumours (Levin, 1976). Vincristine with its high molecular weight may not penetrate into the periphery of the tumour where the active growing edge of the tumour lies, because of a partially intact blood brain barrier.

The present study indicates that the the length of relapse free interval in patients, with malignant glioma, undergoing chemotherapy is linked with in-vitro sensitivity to PCB and or CCNU and that this relationship is not due to imbalances in prognostic factors between sensitive and insensitive patients.

ACKNOWLEDGEMENTS

The authors would like to thank Miss E.A. Paul of the Statistics
and Computing Centre, Institute of Neurology, for invaluable help
with the statistical analysis. The work is supported by the
Brain Research Trust and the Cancer Research Campaign.

REFERENCES

Alberts, D., S. Leigh, E. Surwit, R. Serokman, T. Moon and S.
Salmon (1984) In "Human Tumor Cloning" eds Salmon, S. and Trent,
J., Grune-Stratton, Orlando, 509-519.

Barranco, S., B. Drewinko and R. Humphrey (1973) Mutation Res.
19, 277-280.

Barranco, S., D. Ho, B. Drewinko, M. Romsdahl and R. Humphrey
(1972) Cancer Res. **32**, 2733-2736.

Barranco, S., B. Haenelt and E. Gee (1978) Cancer Res. **38**, 656-
660.

Biorklund, A., L. Hakansson, B. Stenstam, C. Trope and M. Akerman
(1980) Eur. J. Cancer **16**, 647-654.

Dendy, P. (1981) Arch. Geschwulstforsch. **51**, 111-118.

Dexter, D., E. Spremulli, Z. Fligiel, J. Barbosa, R. Vogel, A.
van Voorhees and P. Calabresi (1981) Am. J. Med. **71**, 949-956.

Dexter, D., H. Kowalski, B. Blazar, Z. Fligiel, R. Vogel, and G.
Heppner (1978) Cancer Res. **38**, 3174-3181.

Durie, B., L. Young and S. Salmon (1983) Blood **61**, 929-934.

Hakansson, L. and C. Trope (1974a) Acta Pathol. Microbiol. Scand.
A. **82**, 35-40.

Hakansson, L. and C. Trope (1974b) Acta Pathol. Microbiol. Scand.
A. **82**, 41-47.

Heppner, G., D. Dexter, T. DeNucci, F. Miller and P. Calabresi
(1978) Cancer Res. **38**, 3758-3763.

Kornblith, P., B. Smith and L. Leonard (1981) Cancer **47** 255-265.

Kornblith, P. and P. Szypko (1978) J. Neurosurg. **48**, 580-586.

Levin, V. (1976) Advances in Neurology **15**, 315-325.

Limburg, H. and U. Heckmann (1968) J. Obstet. Gynaecol. Br.
Cwlth. **75**, 1246-1255.

Lotan, R. (1979) Cancer Res. **39**, 1014-1019.

Morgan, D., R. Freshney, J. Darling, D. Thomas and F. Celik (1983) Br. J. Cancer **47**, 205-214.

Rosenblum, M., M. Gerosa, C. Wilson, G. Barger, B. Pertuiset, N. de Tribolet and D. Dougherty (1983) J. Neurosurg. **58**, 170-176.

Salmon, S., A. Hamburger, B. Soehnlen, B. Durie, D. Alberts and T. Moon (1978) New Engl. J. Med. **298**, 1321-1327.

Siracky, J. (1979) Br. J. Cancer **39**, 570-577.

Thomas, D., J. Darling, R. Freshney and D. Morgan (1979) In "Multidisciplinary Aspects of Brain Tumor Therapy. eds Paoletti, P. et al. Elsevier/North Holland Biomedical Press, 19-35.

Thomas, D., J. Darling, E. Paul et al. (1985) Br. J. Cancer **51**, 525-532.

Trope, C., K. Aspergren, S. Kullander and B. Astedt (1979) Acta Obstet. Gynaecol. Scand. **58**, 543-546.

Trope, C., L. Hakansson and H. Dencker (1975) Neoplasma **22**, 423-430.

Wheeler, T., P. Dendy and A. Dawson (1974) Oncology **30**, 362-376.

PART THREE

TOPICS IN BRAIN TUMOR THERAPY

Stereotactic Biopsy of Brain Lesions

Ch. B. Ostertag

Abteilung für Stereotaktische Neurochirur gie Neurochirurgische
Klinik der Universität des Saarlandes, D-6650 Homburg/Saar,
Federal Republic of Germany

ABSTRACT

The morbidity associated with specific treatment (surgery,
radiation, chemotherapy) of brain lesions requires
precise information as to the nature and biology of a
lesion. Stereotactic biopsy in its permanent form offers
a logical and reliable guidance for the choice of
treatment.

KEYWORDS

Brain tumor biopsy; stereotactic techniques; neuropathology; brain tumor classification; computed tomography.

INTRODUCTION

Even today's refined neuro-imaging techniques cannot provide
a histological diagnosis. A histological diagnosis - by
definition - can only be made from the examination of a
tissue specimen through a microscope and this is where the
stereotactic biopsy has its primary objective.

CT - STEREOTACTIC BIOPSY

A whole new situation for stereotactic surgery was certainly
created by the diagnostic potential of high resolution
computed tomography (CT) and magnetic resonance, along with
the technique of creating highly detailed images in any
conceivable plane. Both imaging-techniques contain a body of
three-dimensional information which is used for stereotactic target definition. By incorporating angiography into
the stereotactic system, the neurosurgeon has a complete

three-dimensional image of the vascular and the structural
details of individual brain.
There is a wide variety of CT-adapted stereotactic
instruments, each of which has advantages and disadvantages.
RIECHERT's (1951) stereotactic system* is used at this
institution. The headring of the stereotactic system is
mounted on the patient's skull with four metal screws.
The patient is then brought to a CT-scanner**. The ring is
clamped to the CT-table with a specially designed ring
holder. The clamps hold the ring securely parallel to the
scanning plane of the CT-gantry. Since the stereotactic
apparatus uses rectilinear coordinates for indexing, we can
transfer the coordinates from the CT-scanner without making
any modifications. After CT-scanning, the patient is taken
back to the stereotactic operating room. The routine clinical
work at the CT-scanner can go on undisturbed. Biopsy and the
implantation of radioisotopes are generally carried out under
local anaesthesia using a mild sedative medication. The
routine procedure takes about 1 - 1 1/2 hours including
positioning of the patient, X-rays etc. The patient is
allowed to leave the bed the same evening, as there is
usually no major discomfort or brain trauma.

Tissue samples are taken stepwise in distances of 3-5
millimeter ("serial biopsy") using specially designed biopsy
forcepses*** which have a shaft diameter of 1.0 and 1.4
millimeter respectively. The amount of tissue of each sample
is approximately one to four cubic millimeter. The number of
samples varies according to the size of the lesion. The
biopsy is carried out in every brain compartment, the
functionally critical cortical areas included. In clinical
practice we first make an intraoperative smear preparation
diagnosis. Further samples are processed for embedding and
routine stains including semi-thin sections. The method of
staining and the examination of the smear under microscope,
which is achieved within minutes, is described in a previous
paper (OSTERTAG et al., 1980). Tumor nomenclature and grading
is performed according the WHO - tumor classification (ZÜLCH,
1979). Usually the neuropathologist is in the operating area,
so that we are able to discuss together all the details of
the individual case, such as the duration of anamnesis,
major symptoms, angiographic and CT-features.

---

*   Riechert stereotactic system manufactured by F.L.
        Fischer, 7800 Freiburg, West Germany

**   Somatom DR manufactured by Siemens AG,
        8520 Erlangen, West-Germany

***   Biopsy forceps manufactured by F.L. Fischer,
        7800 Freiburg, West-Germany

RESULTS

Since the opening of the department one year ago (April 1984
through May 1985) 196 patients underwent a stereotactic
diagnostic brain biopsy. The majority of lesions (62 %) were
located in functionally critical areas, i.e. mostly fronto-
temporal, insular or in the central region. The remaining
were located in the basal ganglia-thalamus (16 %), midbrain-
pons (13 %) and suprasellar-hypothalamic region (9 %).
79 % of the lesions proved to be neoplastic, 11 % were of
developmental origin, 8 % of vascular origin and 2 % infectious.

The tumors most frequently found (48 %) were astrocytomas
Grade I - III (WHO). It is understood, however, that this
series is composed of patients, who were primarily considered either poor candidates for open surgery or candidates
for radiotherapy. The type of appropriate subsequent
treatment was teletherapy in 75 cases (48 %), brachytherapy
in 28 cases (18 %), craniotomy and resection in 14 cases
(10 %), and a wait-and-see attitude in 25 cases (14 %). The
contents of cystic lesions (14 cases) can be evacuated and
permanently drained off. This especially applies to colloid
cysts, solitary cystic craniopharyngiomas and arachnoid cysts
in which cases the stereotactic procedure can achieve a
definitive treatment (Ostertag et al., 1981; Moringlane and
Ostertag, 1985).

COMPLICATIONS

In our small series we had two mortalities. One was a
65-year-old woman with a frontal glioblastoma. She died
after a generalized seizure, the third day after the
biopsy. The second mortality was due to a hemorrhage in a
basal ganglia metastasis. Looking through the literature, one
finds that the rate of transient complication is now, in the
major series, within the range of 3 %. The mortality,
however, has considerably decreased and is now around 1 % or
below (PECKER et al., 1979; OSTERTAG et al., 1980; EDNER,
1981; SEDAN et al., 1981; MUNDINGER 1982; BOSCH et al., 1982;
BROGGI et al., 1983; DE DEVITIIS et al., 1983; SEDAN et al.,
1984; WILLEMS et al., 1984; APPUZZO et al., 1984; COLOMBO et
al., SCERATTI et al., 1984; KELLY et al., 1984;   MONSAINGEON
et al., 1984).

DISCUSSION

We now use the WHO-system for the classification of brain
lesions. This WHO-grading system means a major change of
course for neuropathology, since it incorporates the clinical
malignancy of a given tumor. The old grading systems were
based solely on the morphology of a tumor. These

morphological features include the increase of cellularity,
the presence and rate of mitotic figures, the presence of
atypical mitotic figures, pleomorphism of tumor cells,
pleomorphism of tissue architecture, in particular, necroses,
stromal reaction, and overgrowth and the formation of
pathological blood vessels. However, what was evident was
that these features, which are generally regarded as signs of
malignancy, do not necessarily indicate malignancy in the
case of tumors of the central nervous system. The best
example is the morphology of the oligodendroglioma, which
clinically is a relatively benign tumor, but which
morphologically has all features of a malignant lesion.

Consequently, the new WHO-grading system was based on a
retrospective assessment of the postoperative prognosis and
survival rates of other known similar examples, i.e. the
biology of these tumor entities was taken into account
(ZÜLCH, 1979).

Many neurosurgeons and neuropathologists not familiar with
the stereotactic techniques have major objections to the
method: the biopsy probes are too tiny for histological
processing, the sampling is not representative of the tumor,
there is a risk of bleeding. KLEIHUES et al. (1984) have
compiled a series of 600 stereotactic biopsies to gather data
on the diagnostic potential and the accuracy of the method.
They found that the smear preparation and the paraffin
embedded sections together provided a definite tumor diagnosis, including tumor type and approximate grading in
82%. In an additional 11 %, a clinically suspected neoplastic
lesion was ruled out by the combination of procedures. That
means that the overall diagnostic potential is more than
90%. In 4.5 % a glioma was diagnosed, but precise grading was
not possible. In the remaining cases, the presence of a tumor
was confirmed, but the tissue samples were insufficient for
histopathological classification. This was, of course, a
retrospective analysis based on autopsy cases, on material
from craniotomies, and, in the majority of cases on patient
follow-up studies. Correlating the cytologic diagnosis
obtained from the smear preparation and the paraffin section
diagnosis, they found that the methods corresponded in 77 %.
There was no correlation in 10.5 %, no discrepancy and no
confirmation in 12.5 %. These figures correspond well with
other published data on stereotactic serial biopsies (EDNER,
1981; DE DIVITIIS et al., 1983; WILLEMS et al., 1984; COLOMBO
et al., 1984; MONSAINGEON et al., 1984; SEDAN et al., 1984).
There are some major problems associated with the
histological evaluation of the biopsy. Neoplasms with a
homogenous tissue architecture, such as pilocytic
astrocytomas or germinomas pose no problems. However, in
tumors with varying tissue components, like anaplastic
gliomas or teratoid tumors, the small sample size was, in
several cases, the cause of a diagnostic error. In larger
hemispheric gliomas, the sample size can be increased by
using a larger forceps or device like the one designed by
SEDAN (1981). The distinction between reactive gliosis and
the infiltration zone of gliomas constitutes another
difficulty which, however, is not confined to stereotactic
samples (DAUMAS-DUPORT et SZIKLA, 1981). Perhaps the

considerable progress which has been made in the use of
immunohistochemical techniques for the location of cell and
tumor markers will soon solve these problems. Equally as
important as the morphological diagnosis is the accurate
estimation of the borders of a tumor for the calculation of
tumor volumes when subsequent interstitial radiotherapy is
employed (OSTERTAG, this volume). Beyond routine histological
evaluation tissue samples can be used for cell culture
studies (THOMAS et al., 1984).

In summary, stereotactic biopsy in its present form, which
takes full advantage of the three-dimensional information
provided by CT and MR, can be considered a safe procedure
compared with open craniotomy or free-hand needle biopsy. The
diagnostic potential is in the range of more than 90 %. The
procedure entails a minimal brain trauma, i.e. the integrity
of the brain is preserved. In a number of cases the
stereotactic approach offers the possibility of a definitive
therapy, as in cases of cystic lesions such as colloid cysts,
cystic craniopharyngeomas and arachnoid cysts. At present
there is no excuse for not establishing a histological
diagnosis prior to any invasive and potentially noxious
therapy.

Acknowledgement: This study is supported in part by the
Deutsche Krebshilfe e.V., Bonn (M 37/84/Os 1)

References

Apuzzo, M.L.J., P.T. Chandrasoma, V. Zelman, S.L. Giannotta,
M.H. Weiss (1984). Neurosurgery 15, 502-508.
Bosch D.A., E.J. Ebels, L. Vencken, J.J.A. Mooijen,
J.W.F. Beks (1982). Ned. T. Geneesk. 126, 1765-1770.
Broggi G., A. Franzini, F. Migliavacca, A. Allegranza
(1983). Child's Brain 18, 92-98.
Broggi G., A. Franzini, C. Giorgi, A. Allegranza (1984).
Acta Neurochir., Suppl. 33, 211-212.
Colombo F., L. Casentini, A. Benedetti, F. Pozza,
L. Peserico (1984). Min. Med. 75, 1327-1331.
Daumas-Duport C. and G. Szikla (1981). Neurochirurgie 27,
273-284.
DeDivitiis E., R. Spaziante, P. Cappabianca, F. Caputi,
G. Pettinato, M. Del Basso De Caro (1983).
Appl. Neurophysiol. 46, 295-303.
Edner G. (1981). Acta Neurochir. 57, 213-234.
Kelly P.J., B.A. Kall, S.G. Goerss (1984). Acta Neurochir.,
Suppl. 33, 233-235.
Kleihues P., B. Volk, J. Anagnostopoulos, M. Kiessling
(1984). Acta Neurochir., Suppl. 33, 171-181.
Monsaingeon V., C. Daumas-Duport, M. Mann, S. Miyahara,
G. Szikla (1984). Acta Neurochir., Suppl. 33, 195-200.
Moringlane J.R., C.B. Ostertag (1985). Neurochirurgie,
in press.
Mundinger F. (1982). In: Tumors of the Central Nervous
System in Infancy and Childhood. Voth D., P. Gutjahr,
C. Langmaid C. (eds.), Springer, Berlin-Heidelberg,
pp. 234-246.
Ostertag C.B., H.D. Mennel, M. Kiessling (1980). Surg.
Neurol. 14, 275-283.
Ostertag C.B., F. Mundinger, K. Weigel (1981). Med. et
Hyg. 39, 1994-2008.
Pecker J., J.M. Scarabin, B. Vallee, J.M. Brucher (1979).
Surg. Neurol. 12, 341-348.
Riechert T., M. Wolff (1951). Arch. Psychiat. Z. Neurol.
186, 225-230.
Scerrati M., G.F. Rossi (1984). Acta Neurochir., Suppl. 33,
201-205.
Sedan R., J.C. Peragut, Ph. Farnarier, J. Hassoun,
T. Torres (1981). Neurochirurgie 27, 285-286.
Sedan R., J.C. Peragut, Ph. Farnarier, J. Hassoun,
M. Sethian (1984). Acta Neurochir., Suppl. 33, 207-210.
Thomas D.G,T., J.L. Darling, B.A. Watkins, M.C. Hine
(1984). Acta Neurochir., Suppl. 33, 243-246.
Willems J.G.M.S., J.M. Alva-Willems (1984).
Acta Cytologica 28, 243-248.
Zülch K.J. (1979). World Health Organization, Pub. No. 21,
Geneva.

Telethermy and Lasers in the Treatment of Glioblastoma Multiforme

F. Heppner*, St. Schuy**, P. W. Ascher*,
P. Holzer* and G. Wießpeiner**

*Department of Neurosurgery, Karl-Franzens-University,
Graz, Austria
**Institute of Biomedical Engineering, Graz, Austria

KEYWORDS

Prevention of recurrence of glioblastoma multiforme - Heat deposite in the brain-Induction generator - Carbon Dioxide Laser - Neodymium-YAG-Laser.

INTRODUCTION

The glioblastoma multiforme occupies a special position among tumours of the brain being one of the most frequently found gliomas, relatively easy to operate but always recurring within a short period of time. An unfortunate fact well known to each of us.

The classical treatment consists of exstirpation of the growth, followed by additional therapeutic measures including radiotherapy, which in our experience is of limited but undoubted importance. Permanent remissions after this treatment are so rare that histological mistakes are likely. Therefore, the follow-up of those so-called glioblastomas deserves a particularly critical judgment.

Patients who were operated at an early stage frequently return to their normal life with family, profession and sports seemingly cured. It is all the more depressing when within only one year or so the first faint signs of the recurrence are noticed.

For any neurosurgeon who in view of these facts does not straight away resign research into the treatment of this tumour will constitute a lifelong challenge.

MATERIAL AND METHODS

Of the 1366 patients with a glioma operated at our neurosurgical unit, 521 patients (i.e. 38,14 %) were found to suffer from this malicious complaint (Table 1), by which figures the actuality of our topic is emphasized.

Universitätsklinik für Neurochirurgie Graz

1950 - April 1985 GLIOMAS OF THE BRAIN		n = 1366
GLIOBLASTOMA MULTIFORME	521	38,14 %
ASTROCYTOMA I - IV	431	31,55 %
OLIGODENDROGLIOMA	58	4,25 %
SPONGIOBLASTOMA	68	4,98 %
EPENDYMOMA	65	4,76 %
MEDULLOBLASTOMA	78	5,71 %
UNCLASSIFIED	145	10,61 %
	1366	100 %

Table 1

Table 2 demonstrates our various therapeutic attempts and methods, two of which are to be dealt with in detail.

Univ.-Klinik für Neurochirurgie Graz

COMBINED OPERATIVE TREATMENT OF GLIOBLASTOMA MULTIFORME

Method	Year of Introduction	Published
Intracerebral Co^{60}	1956	Heppner, Kahr (1958)
Cytostatics - Intracerebral*)	1958	Heppner (1959,1962,1963); Heppner,Diemath (1963,1963,1967)
- Intracarotid*)	1960	Heppner, Diemath, Jenkner (1961)
Bacterial Oncolysis *)	1965	Heppner,Möse (1966); Heppner,Möse,Propst (1967); Heppner,Möse (1978); Ascher, Heppner,Möse,Walter (1983)
Plus Antimitotics *)	1966	Heppner,Diemath (1970)
Local heating by intracerebral metal plus high frequency irradiation	1967	Heppner,Schuy,Küttner,Wach (1972); Heppner,Küttner (1975, 1975); Heppner,Wiesspeiner,Schuy,Hasler (1978); Heppner Wiesspeiner (1980); Heppner,Ascher,Holzer,Lanner,Wiess- peiner (1984)
CO_2-Laser *)	1976	Heppner (1977)
- plus metal	1980	Heppner (1981)
Neodymium-YAG-Laser *)	1982	

*) plus Radiotherapy

LOCAL HEATING

In 1965 KERSTING drew our attention to the fact that glioblastoma cells were destroyed at a temperature of 43 °. Bearing this in mind the expectation was justyfied that a periodic generation of heat within the postoperative cavity left after the removal of the tumour should inhibit the regrowth of malignant cells. The application of heat had of course to be limited to the former site of the tumour. So, the task was to procedure a local heat deposite in the cerebrum.

This is to be achieved by utilizing the generation of heat within a high frequency fluctuating magnetic field. The plan was the following: After removal of the tumour, before the wound was closed, the walls of the cavity are lined with a small grained metal powder (Fig. 1 and 2).

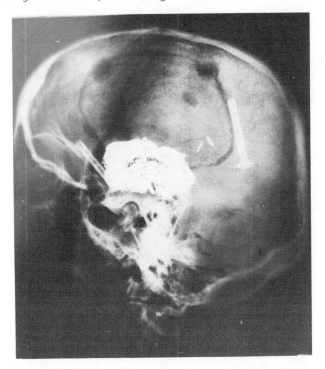

Fig. 1: Metal powder in the tumour cavity of the frontal lobe (lateral view).

Two months later the head of the patient was to be placed (for three periods of 20 sec.) into an electromagnetic field resulting in the inductive heating of the metal powder, destroying all malignant cells along the border metal-brain. The basic physics were simple. Not so the practical realisation. Initially a metal tolerated by without causing damage to the brain tissue had to be found. The particle size was critical: Small enough to adhere to the walls of the tumour cavity, but again large enough to allow the generation of the heat required. Tantalum, silver and nickel were tried in various particle sizes, recently also Iron. Another difficulty was, that low parameters, giving good results in small animals did in no ways correspond to those required in human dimensions. To this purpose a completely new type of condensor as well as an apropriately shaped coil had to be conceived and developed. The effectiveness of the concept was initially tested on models simulating the human head and blood flow. Later tests were conducted on anaesthesized pigs before finally the method proved safe enough for human application. In February 1979 the first patient was thus treated. Since then this procedure is routinely carried out in those patients where the Glioblastoma could be totally removed. 92 patients have so far undergone treatment, 38 with Tantalum, 5 with Silver, 40 with Nickel, 9 with Ferrit. Every 6 weeks the head of these patients is placed into the electromagnetic field for a further course of treatment.

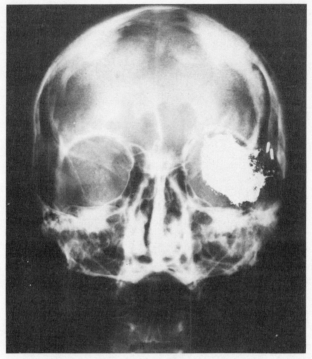

Fig.2: Metal powder in the tumor cavity of the frontal lobe (a.p. view).

TECHNIQUE AND DETAILS

After experimental studies and implantation of different metal powders (Tantalum Nickel,Silver),we found out a compound of ferrite and silver. Characteristic of this implant is optimal warming and good biocompatibility, but production technology is fairly complicated, as mentioned above.

A particle size of 500 microns proofed to be a good compromise between sufficient warming and adhesion on the wound (i.e. cavity   wall).

Like the implant a special induction generator was constructed at the Institute of Biomedical Engineering (TU Graz) (Fig. 3).

The power induction circuit delivers up to 400 Ampères through the special formed application coil and compensation capacitor. At these high currents water cooling inside the wires of power components is necessary.

The peculiar form of the   induction coil (Fig. 4 + 5) renders it possible to deliver a nearly homogenous magnetic field that reaches all regions of the brain with a sufficient field strength (4 kAm^{-1} at 8 MHz). Although a voltage of 3500 V is used in the direct vicinity of the patients head, safety is garanteed by careful isolation.

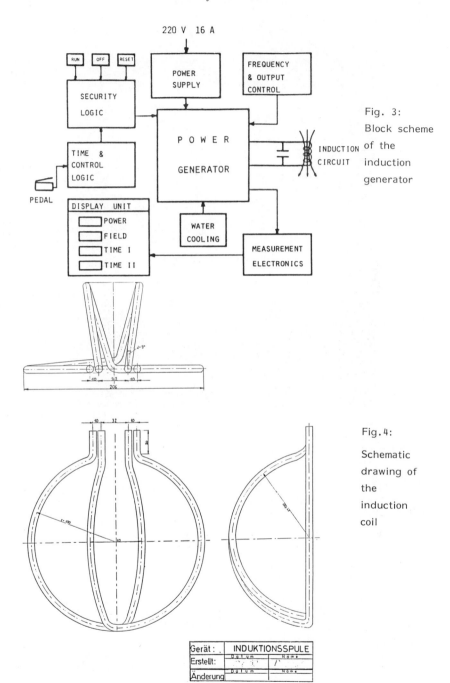

Fig. 3:
Block scheme of the induction generator

Fig. 4:

Schematic drawing of the induction coil

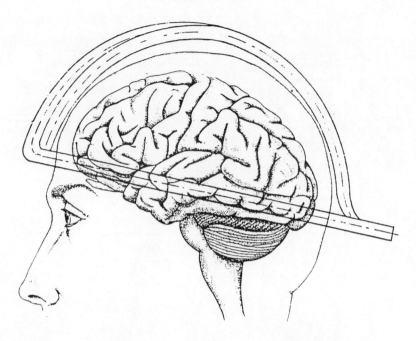

Fig. 5: Placing the Coil on the Patients Head aims at the
         Former Tumours Bed.

At intervals of several weeks the patient is called for hyperthermic session.
This is a very easy treatment. Duration of field and pause time are preselected
on the induction unit. The patients head is placed into the coil centered to
the tumour area (Fig. 6). A pedal switch causes the HF-generator to turn
on producing the magnetic field. The timer circuits automatically control
treatment and pause time. Actual time and field values are displayed.

Depending on the patients recovery (determined by a CT) at one session we
normally perform three magnetic inductions of 30 seconds with an interval of
60 seconds. After this treatment of totally less than five minutes the patient
leaves on his own.

RESULTS

From 92 patients treated this way, 63 have relapsed despite the treatment, the
fate of 15 is unknown but 16 have survived for more than 3 years. The
number of 7 patients, in whom silvered Ferrit was implanted, is as yet too
small and above all, the period too short for any statistical deductions. Some
patients needed a second operation because of tumour recurrence (ca.40%) or
allergy (ca.30% with the formerly used nickel powder). Facing these
figures we feel that for the first time in de depressing and unsatisfactory
history of the treatment of glioblastoma, a cautious optimism seems to be
justified.

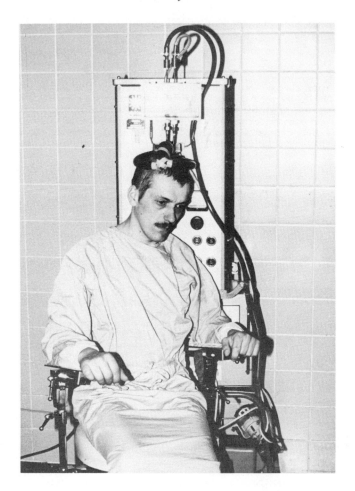

Fig.6: Therapeutic Periodical Session After Operation.

CO_2-LASER

1976 we introduced together with ASCHER for the first time a CO_2-Laser beam into neurosurgical operative technique (Fig. 7). As an instrument which particularly protects the adjacent tissue, it not only serves to remove a tumour, but, most important, using a defocussed beam it allows vaporisation of the tumour bed, meaning a high temperature degradation of the cellular protein along the walls of the tumor cavity.

In this way we hoped to destroy invisible remaining tumour cells. However of the more than 177 patients treated with this method (Table 3) our hopes were fullfilled in a few cases only. All others relapsed within one and a half year.

Since 1982 vaporisation is carried out with the Neodymium-YAG-Laser but time is yet too short to venture an assessment. There is no doubt, that using the Neodymium-YAG-Laser, due to its greater depth of penetration, its scattering within the tissue a wider margin of the tumour bed is covered.

SUMMARY

Summarizing it may be stated that nowadays the combination of local hyper-thermia with laser surgery is carried out as a routine in those cases in which glioblastoma multiforme or a grade IV astrocytoma could be completely exstirpated. In contrast, this method is obviously useless in those cases were only a partial removal is performed. Regardless these new attempts no changes in the primary hypothetical immuno biological situation underlying the regrowth of the glioblastoma may be expected.

Laser Operations carried out at the "Universitätsklinik

für Neurochirurgie in Graz"

June 28th 1976 - June 28th 1984

GLIOBLASTOMAS 177
ASTROCYTOMAS 122
MENINGIOMAS 91
METASTASIS 85
OTHERS 92

            TUMORS OF THE PINEAL GLAND 9
            ADENOMAS OF THE PITUITARY GLAND .6
            PLEXUS PAPILLOMAS 3
            MEDULLOBLASTOMAS 15
            CRANIOPHARYNGEOMAS 5
            ACOUSTIC NERVE TUMOURS 10
            ANGIOMAS & AVM 16
            EPENDYMOMAS 24
            TUMOURS OF THE CORPUS CALLOSUM.. 4

OTHERS, NON CLASSIFIED TUMORS 17
OTHERS INTRACRANIAL PROCESSES 37

            HEMORRHAGIC CYSTS 18
            ARACHNOIDAL CYSTS 6
            ABSCESSES 5
            TUBERCULOMAS 1
            PROCEDURES ON EPILEPTICS 7

OPERATIONS OF THE SPINAL CORD 35

            EXTRAMEDULLARY TUMOURS 21
            INTRAMEDULLARY TUMOURS 10
            FUNCTIONAL SURGERY 4

OPERATIONS ON PERIPHERAL NERVES 28
CRANIOSTENOSIS 4
DIVERSES 52

        Totall Number of Operations with Laser   756

        Operations with CO_2-Laser   643

        Operations with Nd:YAG-Laser   113

have been carried out at the University Clinic of Neuro-
                surgery at Graz,
                    AUSTRIA

Table 3

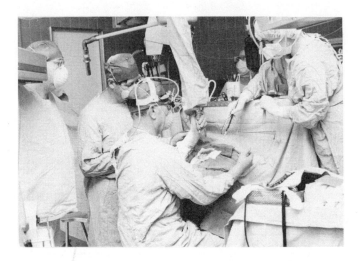

Fig.7: Brain operation with the Carbon Dioxide Laser.
Note the distance between the handpiece and the brain
surface ("Non-touch technique").

REFERENCES

Ascher, P.W. (1976). Der CO_2-Laser in der Neurochirurgie. Molden (Vienna).
Heppner, F. and Ascher, P.W. (1976). Acta Medicotechn. 24, 424-426.
Heppner, F. and Ascher, P.W. (1977). Acta Chir. Austriaca 9/2, 32-34.
Heppner, F. , Ascher, P.W. et al. (1984). Proceedings Medizin und Technik
    19.5.1984 (Graz).
Heppner, F. (1984). Proceedings Congress of the Scandinavian Neurosurgical
    Society, Stockholm, Sept. 13th. Special Lecture.
Kersting, G. (1965). Personal Communication.
Küttner, J., Schuy, St. and Heppner, F. (1973). "E und M" 90/4, 176-180.
Schuy, St., Küttner, J., Wach, P. and Heppner, F. (1972). Biomed. Techn.17,
    74-80, 1972.

Methodology of Serial Stereotactic Biopsy of Glial Tumors

G. Broggi, A. Franzini, C. Giorgi and
A. Allegranza

Department of Neurosurgery, Istituto Neurologico "C. Besta",
Milano, Italy

KEY WORDS

Glial Tumors; Stereotactic biopsy; Computerized Tomography (C.T.); Nuclear Magnetic Resonance (N.M.R.).

INTRODUCTION

Nowadays the histological diagnosis of glial tumors cannot be considered the only final goal of stereotactic biopsy; much more data about the tumor must be provided by this stereotactic procedure in order to investigate the volume of the lesion, the neurophysiological relationships with surrounding tissue, the modalities of neoplastic growth, the proliferative activity and other prognostic indices (Broggi et al., 1983).
All these data may represent the starting point to assess the indications and to evaluate the effectiveness of old and new therapeutic techniques including ablative and conservative treatments. The multimodal approach to this stereotactic method is mandatory , in our opinion, to study the relationships between the neuroradiological images and the real extension and structure of glial tumors with particular reference to the Computerized Tomography (C.T.) and to the Nuclear Magnetic Resonance (N.M.R.).
The full procedure of stereotactic biopsy is described and the value of intra-operative neurophysiological assessment and multiple tissues sampling is stressed. The significance of the definitive results is related to the rightness of each single operative item.

METHODS

Different stereotactic apparatus may be used to perform correct stereotactic biopsies; the currently utilized systems include the Talairach frame (Talairach et al., 1967) the Todd Wells frame (Todd, 1967), the Leksell frame (Leksell,

1949; Leksell and Jernberg, 1980), the Riechert frame (Riechert and Mundinger,
1957) and the Brown Roberts frame (Brown, 1979); the last two apparatus have
been utilized for stereotactic biopsy in our Department and the procedure of
deep brain biopsy described in the following paragraphs may be easy accomplished
by all these systems following the same procedural items.

A - Transposition of C.T. and N.M.R. images in the stereotactic space. Since
    the stereotactic apparatus provides lateral and frontal radiographies of the
    skull, the C.T. and N.M.R. images of the lesion may be transferred in these
    planes by simple mathematical proocedures (Gildenberg and Kaufman, 1982);
    the mathematical transposition is made easier when the scout view of the
    C.T. examination is available. Direct transposition between C.T. and
    stereotactic X rays may be performed by C.T. dedicated or C.T. adapted
    stereotactic frames (Cohadon et al., 1977; Kelly et al., 1979; Apuzzo and
    Sabshin, 1983).
    The ideal method to localize the tumor in the stereotactic space should be
    the use intraoperative C.T. examinations in stereotactic conditions and
    assisted by computer graphic technology; encouraging experimental results in
    this field have been recently obtained in our Department (unpublished data).
    To confirm the localization of the tumor, ventriculography may be performed
    in stereotactic conditions and the relationships between the ventricles and
    the lesion allow to verify the previous reconstruction. When indirect
    methods of transposition are utilized, stereotactic ventriculography is
    mandatory.

B - Stereotactic carotid angiography is performed when the target lesion is
    seated within the temporal lobe: in these cases the trajectory is calculated
    in order to avoid the vascular structure of the Sylvian region (Szikla et
    al., 1981). Intraoperative angiography is also needed when major vessels
    displacement is demonstrated by preoperative examinations. Deep seated
    tumors within the basal ganglia, the brainstem and hemispheric white matter,
    usually do not require intraoperative angiography as in stereotactic
    procedures performed for abnormal movements or intractable pain (thalamo-
    tomy, tractotomy, pallidotomy). Out of 227 stereotactic biopsies performed
    in patients affected from glial tumors, 87 cases underwent stereotactic
    intraoperative carotidography. Preoperative angiography by conventional or
    digital technique has been performed in all patients. Advances in digital
    technology will allow the complete tridimensional evaluation of cerebral
    vessels in stereotactic condition in order to choice the riskless trajectory
    to the lesion; preliminary results in this field have been recently obtained
    in our Department (unpublished data). Digital stereotactic angiography,
    intraoperative C.T. and intraoperative N.M.R. in stereotactic conditions
    represent, in our opinion, the opimization of stereotactic surgery (Koslow
    et al., 1981)

C - Impedance monitoring along the full stereotactic trajectory from the cortex
    to the deepest boundaries of the tumor is routinely performed to investigate
    the structural features of the lesion as necrotic areas, cysts and major
    edema of tissues surrounding the tumor (Benabid et al., 1978; Broggi and
    Franzini, 1981). This technique revealed an high accuracy to confirm the
    rightness of the transtumoral trajectory and the impedance profile is
    utilized to choice the series of targets for tissue sampling (Figure 1).

Moreover **in presence of cystic** lesions, the impedance monitoring is utilized to optimize the implant of intracavitary catheters for periodic aspirations or in view of interstitial radiotherapy by radiocolloids (Szikla et al., 1981). The equipment utilized is the RFG5S Radionics apparatus connected to bipolar electrode gently indwelled along the choosen trajectory.

D - Depth EEG recording is perfomed in patients in which epilepsy is the prevailing symptom of the tumor; in most of these cases the lesion detected by C.T. and N.M.R. examinations is poorly definite and appears as shaded hypodense area (Broggi et al., 1984); the neoplastic areas and the peritumoral irritative zones are easy localized by this technique and the sampling of tissues is guided to the areas characterized by slow lesional activity (Laitinen and Toivakka, 1972; Laitinen, 1976) or by so called "electrical silence" (Figure 1). Moreover the localization and the features of epileptic activity are additional data to study the modalities of tumor development. When more complex neurosurgical operations will be performed in term of surgical treatment of epilepsy, much more depth EEG data will be provided and the stereo-EEG performed in three planes is the technique of choice (Bancaud et al., 1973; Sedan, 1976).

E - Intraoperative smear examinations by supravital Methylen Blue staining (Ostertag et al., 1980) is routinely performed on small fragments from each tissue sample and the presence of neoplastic glial cells may confirm intraoperatively the rightness of the procedure; in many cases this technique allows the histological diagnosis (presence of necrotic areas or presence of polymorphic cells suggest the diagnosis of glioblastoma). Moreover in most cases the intraoperative histological examination represents the starting point to plan the sampling of tissues from multiple "strategic" targets along the stereotactic trajectory and in some cases may suggest the need of more trajectories through the tumor and surrounding tissues.

F - Tissue sampling within the choosen targets may be performed by the original Sedan aspiration instrument (Sedan et al. 1975) which provides cylinders of tissue (about 10 millimeters lenght and 1 millimeter diameter) or by the original Backlund instrument (Backlund and Leksell, 1971) which utilizes an inner coil to pick-up the cylinder of tissue. Both these apparatus allow to obtain much more tissue than the biopsy forceps (original Fisher instrument) which are conversely indicated in brain stem lesions to take out small fragments of tissue avoiding the risks of damaging the neuroanatomical structures of this region (Ostertag et al., 1980).
Whatever the utilized instrument, the value of multiple tissue samples within the tumor and within surrounding tissue is stressed (Waltregny et al., 1974).

G - Implant of a small metallic marker at the deepest target within the tumor is the last step of the procedure and allow to assess post-operatively the site of biopsy. The utilized marker must be N.M.R. compatible and usually has been obtained from fragments of haemostatic surgical clips.

Part of the procedure and an exemplificative case is represented in Figure 1.

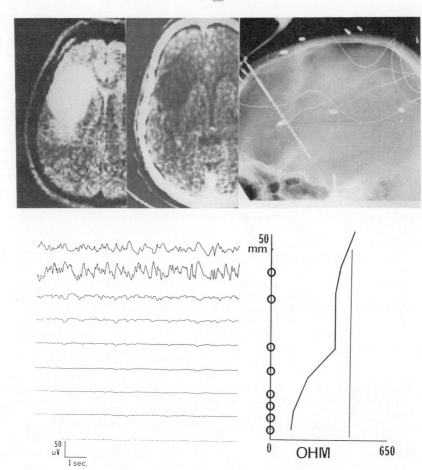

Fig. 1 N.M.R. and C.T. examinations in a 37 years old male
patient affected by left fronto-temporal astrocytoma (upper
left). Depth EEG multipolar electrode inserted along the
stereotactic trajectory within the tumor (upper right).
Depth EEG recording shows slow wave activity and the so
called "electric silence" at the deepest channel while
irritative activity is present on the upper channels which
correspond to the nervous tissues surrounding the lesion
(lower left). Impedance recording at the same levels of the
depth EEG channels shows a decrease corresponding to the
lesional EEG activity; the targets choosen for tissues
sampling are represented by circles on the ordinates line of
the impedance profile (lower right).
The definitive histological diagnosis in this case resulted
mature astrocytoma.

RESULTS AND DISCUSSION

Between January 1978 and April 1984, 227 patients affected from glial tumors underwent serial stereotactic biopsies. The obtained histological diagnosis has been verified in 64 patients which underwent surgical removal of the lesion after biopsy; in the series of patients which underwent conservative therapy, the long term follow-up (1-6 years) has been assumed to confirm or deny the previous histological diagnosis. Correct histological diagnosis and grading (W.H.O., 1979) has been obtained in 193 patients (85% of the whole series); in 24 patients the stereotactic biopsy provided only the diagnosis of nature while the histological grading resulted missed (10.5% of the whole series); finally in 10 patients the target itself resulted missed and no histological diagnosis has been obtaineed (4.5% of the whole series).

The operative mortality included 6 patients (2.6% of the whole series); permanent major neurological deficits occurred in 5 patients (2.2%) and permanent minor neurologica deficit occurred in 4 patients (1.7%).

In conclusion the described methodology allowed positive results in 85% of cases but it need to be continuously improved by computer assisted technology including intraoperative C.T. and N.M.R. examinations, stereotactic digital angiography and tridimensional computerized reconstruction techniques. Moreover the developing of cell kinetic studies to assess the potential proliferative activity of glial tumors will provide much more data to assess the behaviour of gliomas and to plan the correct treatment of these tumors.

REFERENCES

Apuzzo, M.L.J., and J.K. Sabshin (1983). Neurosurgery, 12, 277-285.

Backlund, E., and L. Leksell (1971). Acta Chir. Scand., 137, 825.

Bancaud, J., J. Talairach, S. Geier and J.H. Scarabin (1973). EEG et SEGG dans les tumeurs cérébrales et l'épilepsie. Ediflor Ed., Paris.

Benabid, A.L., J.C. Persat, J.P. Chirossel, J. De Rougemont and M. Barge (1978). Neurochirurgie, 24, 3-14.

Broggi, G., and A. Franzini (1981). J. Neurol. Neurosurg. Psychiatry, 44, 397-401.

Broggi, G., A. Franzini, C. Giorgi, R. Spreafico and G. Avanzini (1984). Acta Neurochir. Suppl. 33, 97-103.

Broggi, G., A. Franzini, A. Costa, A. Melcarne and A. Allegranza (1985). Appl. Neurophysiol., in press.

Brown, R.A. (1979). J. Neurosurg., 50, 715-720.

Cohadon, F., A. Rougier, D. Da Silva Nunes Neto, J. Pigneux, J.M. Caille and P. Constans (1977). Neurochirurgie, 23, 434-452.

Gildenberg, P.L., and H.H. Kaufman (1982). Appl. Neurophysiol., 45, 347-351.

Kelly, P.J., H.O. Marvin, A.E. Wright and C. Giorgi (1979). In Stereotactic Cerebral Irradiation, ed. G. Szikla, Elsevier North Holland, Amsterdam, pp. 123-128.

Koslow, M., M.G. Abele, R.G. Griffith, G.A. Mair and N.E. Chase (1981). Neurosurgery, 8, 72-82.

Laitinen, L. (1976). Ann. Radiol., 19, 237-239.

Laitinen, L., and E. Toivakka (1972). Confin. Neurol., 34, 101-105.

Leksell, L. (1949). Acta Chir. Scand., 99, 229-233,

Leksell, L., and B. Jernberg (1980). Acta Neurochir., 52, 1-7.

Ostertag, C.B., H.D. Mennel and M. Kiessling (1980). Surg. Neurol., 14, 275-283.
Riechert, T., and F. Mundinger (1957). In Introduction to stereotaxy with an atlas of the human brain, Vol.1, eds. B. Schaltenbrand and P. Bailey. G. Thieme, Stuttgart, pp. 437-471.
Sedan, R. (1976). Neurochirurgie, 22, 599-601.
Sedan, R., J.C. Peragut and P. Vallicioni (1975). Présentation d'un appareillage original pour biopsie cérébrale et tumorale en conditions stéréotactiques. Communication à la Société de Neurochirurgie de Langue Française. Decembre.
Szikla, G., O. Betti, L. Szenthe and M. Schienger (1981). Neurochirurgie, 27, 295-298.
Talairach, J., G. Szikla, P. Tournoux, A. Prossalentis. H. Bordas-Ferrer, L. Covello, M. Jacob and E. Mempel (1967). Atlas d'anatomie stéréotaxique du telencéphale. Masson et Cie. Ed., Paris.
Todd, E. M. (1967). Todd-Weels: Manual of streotactic procedures. Codman Shurless, Randolph.
Waltregny, A., V. Petrov and J. Brotchi (1974). Acta Neurochir., 21, 221-226.
W.H.O. (1979). Histological classification of tumors of the nervous system. Geneva.

AKNOWLEDGEMENTS

Thanks are due to M. Bracchi M.D. who conducted the intraoperative stereo-tactic angiography in most cases and to A. Melcarne M.D. who assisted in the preparation of the manuscript. This study has been partially supported by grant n° 84.00474.44 from the Consiglio Nazionale delle Ricerche, Roma, Italy.

Photodynamic Therapy of Brain Tumors: Studies on the Distribution of DHE (Di-Hematoporphyrin Ether) in Normal and Experimental Neoplastic Brain Tissue in Rats

A. Olivi*, M. Waner**, R. Sawaya*,
T. Wesseler***, P. Cassini*, B. Liwnicz***,
M. Pensak** and J. M. Tew Jr.*

*Department of Neurosurgery, University of Cincinnati,
Cincinnati, Ohio 45267, USA
**Department of Otolaryngology & Maxillo-Facial Surgery,
University of Cincinnati, Cincinnati, Ohio 45267, USA
***Department of Pathology, University of Cincinnati,
Cincinnati, Ohio 45267 USA

KEY WORDS: PHOTODYNAMIC THERAPY, BRAIN TUMORS, HEMATOPORPHYRIN
              DERIVATIVE

INTRODUCTION

The encouraging results obtained by photodynamic therapy (PDT) in
the treatment of a number of non-neural tumors (Doughtery, 1978,
1984) have stimulated several investigators to explore its possible
application to the treatment of intracerebral tumors (Perria, 1980,
Laws, 1981, McCulloch, 1984).   This relatively new treatment
modality is based on the properties of substances called photosensitizers, to be preferentially retained by neoplastic tissue
and to generate a cytotoxic reaction when activated by visible
light (Kessel, 1984).

HPD (Hematoporphyrin Derivative), a synthetic mixture of porphyrins,
has been the most commonly used photosensitizer in the past.
Recently Dougherty has isolated what is presumed to be the active
component of the mixutre, DHE (Dihematoporphyrin Ether) (Dougherty,
1985) (Fig. 1).   The absorption spectra of DHE is represented by
five different bands of the visible light ilusstrated by Fig. 2.

All Correspondence to: A. Olivi, M.D.
                          Department of Neurosurgery
                          University of Cincinnati
                          Cincinnati, Ohio 45267

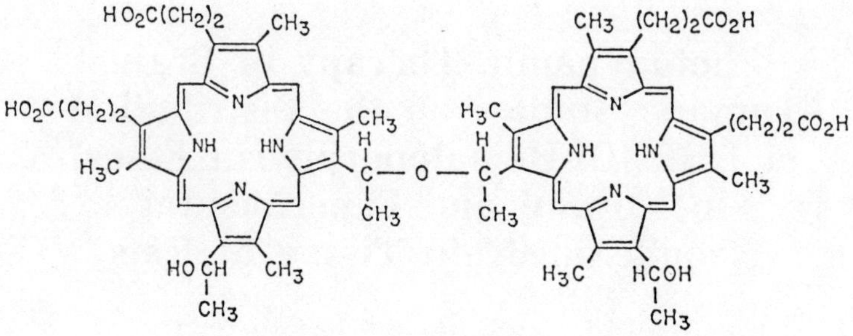

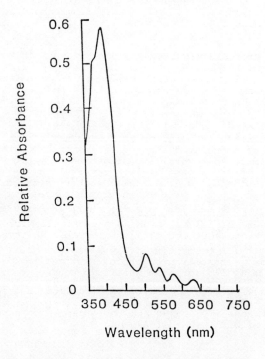

Bis-1-[8-(1-hydroxyethyl)deuteroporphyrin-3-yl]ethyl ether

FIGURE 1. STRUCTURE OF THE ACTIVE COMPONENT
OF HEMATOPORPHYRIN DERIVATIVE.

FIGURE 2. DHE ABSORPTION SPECTRA

Although the maximum absorption occurs at 415 μm, the 630 μm wavelength band is the most commonly used as activating light in in vivo experimental models as well as in clinical application because of its better penetration in tissue ($\sim$1 cm.)(Dougherty, 1985, Kessel, 1984).

Controversial results concerning both the distribution of the photosensitizers and the efficacy of the treatment have been reported in experimental and clinical studies on intracerebral tumors performed to date (Boggan, 1984, Wharen, 1983, Perria, 1980, Laws, 1981, McCulloch, 1984). Our work was designed to present a simple qualitative analysis of the distribution of DHE in normal and neoplastic tissue in rats.

MATERIALS AND METHODS

Normal Brain Study:

16 Wistar rats weighing between 300 and 420 g. were included in this study. 8 rats underwent an intravenous injection of 30 mg/kg of DHE (Photofrin II, Photofrin Med. Inc., Cheektowaga, N.Y.) via the femoral vein. 4 rats were sacrificed by decapitation 4 hours after the injection and 4 rats were sacrificed 24 hours after the injection.   The intracranial contents were excised, immediately frozen (-40°C) and sent for fluorescence microscopy.

Experimental Tumor Study:

A suspension of C6 glioma cells (Benda, 1971) containing 1 x 10^6 cells (20 μl) was injected stereotactically in the left hemisphere of 8 rats. In three of them, a symmetric injection in the right hemisphere of 20 μl of the media alone was performed. 14 days later 30 mg/kg of DHE was injected intravenously.   24 hours after the sensitization, the rats were sacrificed and the intracranial contents excised, frozen and sent for fluorescence microscopy.

Fluorescence Microscopy

The frozen specimens were kept in the dark until the time of examination, which was never later than 2 days after the sacrifice. The specimen were sectioned using a conventional microtome and sequential sections were cut at 4 u intervals. Alternate sections were mounted without fixative and examined with the fluorescence microscope and mounted with fixative, stained using hematoxylin and eosin, and examined with the light microscope.   The fluorescence microscopy was performed using an Olympus Microscope, Model No. BH5, with a reflected light fluorescence attachment No. BH-RFLW.   The excitation light was filtered using an excitor filter Model No. F-490 and the light was viewed through a Barrier Filter with a cut of 420 μm.

RESULTS

Normal Brain Study:

The fluorescence emitted by DHE was bright reddish-orange, distinguishable from the naturally occurring autofluorescence seen in the internal elastic lamina of the blood vessels and in the meninges.

Four hours post injection, an intravascular fluorescence was clearly evident.   Meningeal fluorescence was also present with an uneven distribution (Fig. 3 and Fig. 4).

Twenty-four hours after the injection, the intravascular fluorescence was no longer evident.   The meningeal fluorescence was still present and had become more evenly distributed (Fig. 5 and Fig. 6). No evidence of intracerebral fluorescence was detected in both samples.

Experimental Tumor Study:

The C6 glioma was actively growing 14 days after the implantation as seen in Fig. 7.   In the fluorescence studies, the distribution in the neoplastic tissue was strikingly evident and uniform throughout the extent of the tumor (Fig. 8 and Fig. 9).   No evidence of fluorescence was detected where media was injected alone.   The sharp limits of the fluorescence corresponding to the limits of the tumor were evident in all the samples obtained. In one sample, an infiltration of the tumor into the surrounding normal brain, evident on the H and E slide, can be followed by the fluorescence distribution in the fluorescence microscopy sample (Fig. 10 and Fig. 11).

DISCUSSION

The recent application of photodynamic therapy concepts to the neuro-oncological field has been characterized by a number of controversies regarding the following problems:

1.   The distribution of the photosensitizer in the normal and neoplastic brain tissue.

2.   The potential neurotoxicity.

Wise and Taxdal in 1967 evidenced that hematoporphyrins do not cross the blood-brain barrier in the intact brain.   They were able to detect it in traumatized regions, in the pituitary stalk and in the area postreme (wise, 1967).

Diamond and Granelli first demonstrated the lethal effect of PDT on glioma cells, both cultured and implanted in the subcutaneous tissue of rats, after sensitization with hematoporphyrins (Diamond & Granelli, 1982).   The early clinical studies of Perria, Laws and McCulloch documented a reasonable safety and feasability of PDT in humans (Laws, 1981, Perria, 1980 and McCulloch, 1984). The heterogenity of the clinical material associated with the diversity of the methods used, however, made their results not indicative of the efficacy of the treatment.

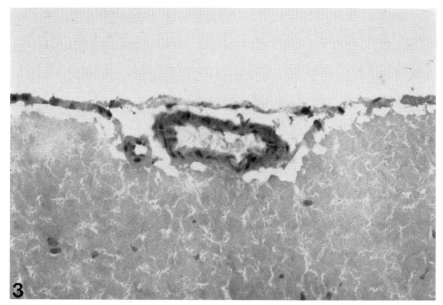

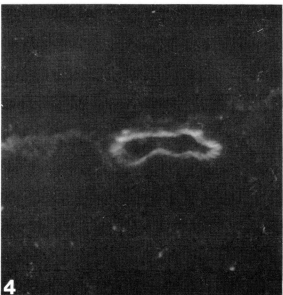

Fig. 3.   An H&E frozen section through the cerebral cortex. Note the presence of a large meningeal vessel, meninges and cortical brain tissue.

Fig. 4.   A similar section 4 hours post i.v. DHE. Note the intravascular plus meningeal fluorescence.

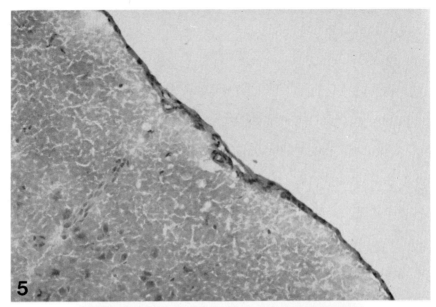

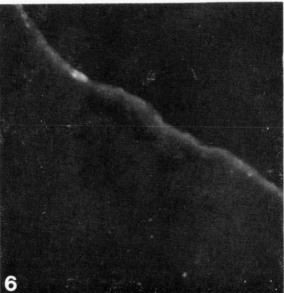

Fig. 5.   An H&E frozen section through the cerebral cortex showing a small meningeal blood vessel, meninges and a section of cerebral cortex.

Fig. 6.   A similar section, 24 hours post i.v. DHE showing meningeal fluorescence. Note absence of cortical fluorescence.

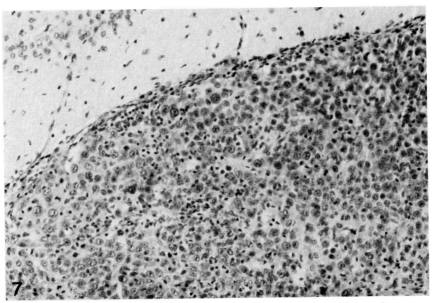

Fig. 7. An H&E paraffin section showing the normal histology of an intracerebral C6 glioma.

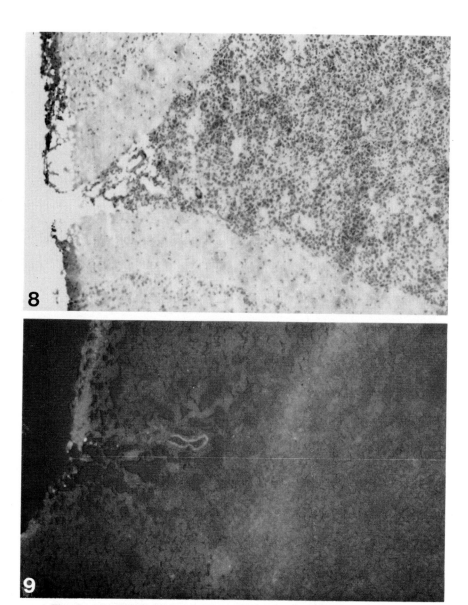

Fig. 8.   An H&E frozen section showing an intracerebral C6 glioma about one week after implantation. Note the meningeal tear made by the passage of the trochar during implantation.

Fig. 9.   A similar section showing intratumoral fluorescence extending right up to the margin of microscopic tumor, but not beyond.

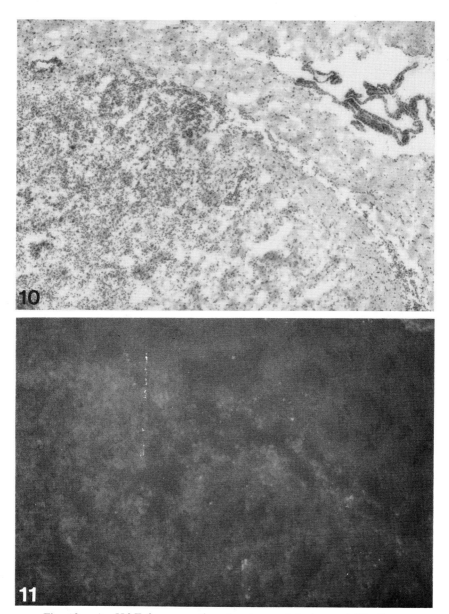

Fig. 10. An H&E frozen section showing an intratumoral C6 glioma.
Note a small area of microscopic spread of the tumor along a tissue plane.

Fig. 11. A similar section showing fluorescence of the tumor as well as
all the areas of microscopic spread.

Other experimental studies evidenced a possible phototoxic involvement of normal brain. Rounds in 1982 and Cheng in 1984 suggested the vulnerability of cerebral tissue of mice and rats respectively, to photodynamic exposure.

Wharen et al confirmed the elevated concentration ratio of hemato-porphyrins between neoplastic tissue and normal brain (Wharen, 1983). Boggan et al indicated, because of the patchy distribution of the photosensitizer in the tumor, a limitation of the effectiveness of PDT (Boggan, et al, 1984).

Our qualitative studies on the distribution of DHE in normal brain have corroborated the hypothesis of the impermeability of an intact blood brain barrier to the hematoporphyrins. Its documented presence in the vascular compartment, however, may represent the possible explanation of the reported neurotoxicity. One of the advocated mechanisms of action of PDT, in fact, is thought to be an indirect tissue   necrosis secondary to vascular damage (Bugelsky, et al, 1981). Studies on the disruption of an intact blood brain barrier after photodynamic exposure would be helpful to confirm this hypothesis.

The clear, unquestionable, uniform distribution of DHE in our C6 experimental gliomas represents, in our opinion, another indication of the variability of the blood brain alteration in different human and experimental tumors.

Since we were not able to detect any fluorescence at the site of the injection of media alone, we think that the extensive uptake of DHE by the neoplastic tissue is a phenomenon strictly related to the intrinsic biological characteristics of the tumor and not a consequence of a mechanical blood brain barrier disruption.

Our results are supportive of the reliability of this model in the study of some of the critical aspects of photodynamic therapy of brain tumors. The extension of the tumor destruction after treatment, the involvement of the surrounding normal brain tissue, the choice of the appropriate light energy and the light delivery system, in fact, need to be investigated to provide further information for a better understanding of this treatment modality, still in its early stages.

REFERENCES

1. Benda, P., Someda, K., Messer, J., Sweet, WH:Morphological and immunochemical studies of rat blial tumors and clonal strains duplicated in culture. J. Neurosurg. 34:310-323, 1971.

2. Boggan, JE., Walter, R., Edwards, SB, Borcich, JK, Davis, RL, Koonce, M., Berns, MW:Distribution of hematoporphyrin derivative in the rat 9Lgliosarcoma brain tumor analyzed by digital video fluorescence in microscopy. J. Neurosurg. 61:1113-1119, 1984.

3. Cheng, MK, McKean, J., Boisvert, D., Tulip, J., Mielke,BW: Effects of photoradiation therapy on normal rat brain. Neurosurgery, Vol. 15, No. 6, 1984.

4. Diamond, I., Granelli, SG, McDonald, AF, et al:Photodynamic therapy of malignant tumors. Lancet 2:117501177, 1982.

5. Bugelsky, PJ., Porter, CW., Dougherty, TS:Autoradiographic distribution of hematoporphyrin derivative in normal and tumor tissue of the mouse. Cancer Res. 41:4606-4612, 1981.

6. Dougherty, TJ:Porphyrin localization and treatment of tumors. P75-87, Alan R. Liss, Inc., 1984.

7. Dougherty, TJ., Potter, WR., Weishaupt, KR:The structure of the active component of hematoporphyrin derivative. Porphyrins in Tumor Phototherapy, Plenum Publishing Corp. P23-35, 1985.

8. Dougherty, TJ, Kaufman, JE., Goldfarb, et al:Cancer Rese. 38:2628-2635, 1978.

9. Kessel, D:Biochem Pharm. 33:1389-1393, 1984.

10. Laws, ER., Cortese, DA., Kinsey, JH., et alPhotoradiation therapy in the treatment of malignant brain tumors:A phase I (Feasability) study. Neurosurg., Vol. 9, No. 6, 1981.

11. McCulloch, GAJ, Forbes, IJ., Lee See, K. et al:Phototherapy of malignant brain tumors in porphyrin localization and treatment of tumors. P709-717, Alan Liss, Inc., 1984.

12. Perria, C., Capuzzo, T., Cavagnaro, G., et al:First attempts at the photodynamic treatment of human gliomas, J. Neurosurg. Sci. 24, p119-129, 1980.

13. Rounds, DE., Jacques, S., Shelden, CH., Shaller, CA., Olson, RS:Development of a protocol for photoradiation therapy of malignant brain tumors:Part 1 Neurosurg. Vol. 11, No. 4, p500, 1982.

14. Wharen, RE., Anderson, RE., Laws, ER:Quantitation of hemato-porphyrin derivative in human gliomas, experimental central nervous system tumors, and normal tissues. Neurosurg. Vol. 12, No. 4, 1983.

15. Wise, BL., Taxdal, DR:Studies of the blood brain barrier utilizing hematoporphyrin. Brain Res. 4, p387-398, 1967

ACKNOWLEDGEMENTS

This project has been conducted with the support of the James N. Gamble Institute of Medical Research and Department of Neurosurgery The Christ Hospital, Cincinnati, Ohio 45219

The authors wish to express gratitude to Drs., Jeffery Keller and Geoffrey M. Thomas for their valuable assistance and Mrs. Kathleen Devanna for her preparation of the manuscript.

Stereotactic Brachytherapy of Brain Tumors

Ch. B. Ostertag

Abteilung für Stereotaktische Neurochirurgie Neurochirurgische
Klinik der Universität des Saarlandes, D-6650 Homburg/Saar,
Federal Republic of Germany

ABSTRACT

In view of the current understanding of the cell
biology of gliomas a conceptual basis for brachytherapy of low grade gliomas using permanent
iodine-125 implants is formed. Biologically, a
local radionecrosis achieves a kinetically significant
reduction of the tumor cellular mass. Animal experiments and clinical experience with patients underscore
the biological advantages of continuous low dose rate
irradiation.

KEYWORDS

Brain Tumor radiation therapy, astrocytoma, brachytherapy, iodine-125, experimental radiation injury.

INTRODUCTION

Treatment of gliomas beyond surgical resection still is
a problem. There has been considerable controversy as to
the value of radiation therapy of gliomas. The benefits
of conventional radiation therapy are limited (KUHLENDAHL
et al., 1973, SCANLON and TAYLOR 1979). External beam
radiation therapy may not only be ineffective but potentially harmful, particularly for long term survivers
(BURGER et al., 1979; SCHIFFER et al., 1980, 1981). Although
occasional brain tumor patients respond remarkably well
to chemotherapy, the majority, however, does not. Irradiation therefore is still the most commonly used treatment
modality. Current radiotherapeutic practice seeks to optimize
therapy by careful definition of the target volume, the
dose distribution and the quality of radiation.
Considerable progress has been made in two areas: more
precise beam techniques (teletherapy) and the placement
of radioactive sources into tumors, i.e. interstitial
radiation therapy (brachytherapy).

175

CONCEPTUAL BASIS OF BRACHYTHERAPY

In conventional radiation therapy, the tolerance of the
healthy brain is critical. This implies a therapeutic
ratio, i.e. a difference in radiosensitivity between
healthy brain and brain tumor tissue. Growth characteristics and mitotic activity of gliomas are major
determinants for the biological effect of therapeutic
radiation. We know from clinical experience that glioblastomas can grow very rapidly and that, on the other
hand, low grade astrocytomas, like cerebellar astrocytomas
or optic chiasm gliomas, grow very slow, if at all. The
studies on the cell kinetics of various gliomas by
HOSHINO et al. (1972) and HOSHINO (1984) have shown
that the labelling index as an indicator for the mitotic
activity is indeed very high in medulloblastomas (12 %)
and glioblastomas (9.3 %), is moderate in anaplastic
astrocytomas and is very low in fibrillary astrocytomas (.8 %). This explains why conventional radiotherapy
is relatively ineffective in tumors with a very low proliferation capacity, and why it is potentially harmful
with respect to late radiation changes (ZEMAN, 1968;
SCHIFFER et al., 1980, 1981; BURGER et al., 1979).

Astrocytomas have a very limited proliferating capacity.
Therefore, in well differentiated gliomas it is important
to remove as much tumor as possible (HOSHINO, 1984; LAWS
et al., 1984). When, however, there is no harmless way of
surgical removal, as in cases of low grade astrocytomas in
the basal ganglia, brainstem, or in functionally critical
cortical areas, radiosurgery in the form of low dose rate
brachytherapy is considered the appropriate treatment modality. Biologically, the local radionecrosis achieves a kinetically significant reduction of the tumor cellular burden.
At present, iodine-125 (I-125) and iridium-192 (Ir-192) are
the most suitable radioisotopes with which to produce a
tumor radionecrosis. Radiation from an interstitially
implanted permanent source such as iodine-125 is continuously delivered at very low dose rates (10-20 cGy/h)
compared with dose rates delivered by external beam. The
therapeutic ratio is enhanced as a result of the rapid
dose fall-off in tissue within a distance of millimeters.
Since radiation from iodine-125 sources is effectively
attenuated by interjacent tissue such as brain, bone of
the skull, and scalp, no special radioprotection is
necessary for either patient or medical personnel.

EXPERIMENTAL BRACHYTHERAPY

How does the normal brain tissue, which is usually involved
in interstitial tumor irradiation, tolerate this radiation?
To study this question, the sequential morphological changes
with permanently implanted iodine-125 and iridium-192
sources in healthy dog brains were observed up to one year
after implantation (OSTERTAG et al., 1982, 1983, 1984;
JANZER et al., 1985). Due to the low photon energy of
iodine-125, much of the energy is absorbed by the tissue
next to the implant. Accordingly, around the implanted
seed we found a necrosis which was always calcified and
which was observed as early as 25 days after the implantation. The size of the necrosis did not increase further
after 70-90 days. The dose which accumulated later apparently did not contribute to the necrotizing effect.
The total size of the necrosis depends on the activity
implanted.

Iridium-192 differs from iodine-125: it has a gamma-
radiation energy which is ten times higher than that of
iodine-125. The iridium-192 implants effected delineated
liquifying and calcifying necrosis. The transitional zone
was characterized by extensive gliosis, which was demonstrated by GFAP positive astrocytes and numerous blood
vessels with an enlarged diameter and thickening of the
vessel wall. Blood vessels with radiation damage could
not be detected in the animals surviving more than 70
days, which means, that blood vessels either were damaged
and incorporated into the necrosis or they were not affected.
Demyelination was always restricted to the ipsilateral
white matter and showed no progression at later stages
of intersitital radiation. In no case did we observe the
the extensive leuko-dystrophic myelin break-down which
occasionally developes as a late complication of external
radiotherapy.

Vasogenic edema, i.e. the permeability changes attributed
to the radionecrosis, was also investigated as a part of
this complex radiolesion having profound clinical implications. For this, we used quantitative autoradiography
with a C-14 alpha-amino-isobutyric acid (OSTERTAG et al.,
1984, GROOTHUIS et al., 1985). This test substance has
many properties which make it ideal for measuring rates
of blood-to-tissue transport. It is a synthetic, inert,
neutral amino acid of low molecular weight that slowly
crosses the blood brain barrier. It is taken up rapidly
by brain cells but is not metabolized and therefore can
serve as an ideal tracer of unidirectional transport
for radiation-induced capillary permeability disturbance
(BLASBERG et al., 1983). In all of the dogs, regardless
of time of exposure, which ranged from 7-717 days, we
found a clearly demarcated sphere of blood brain barrier
break down around the implant, which can persist for over
one year following insertion of the I-125 seed.

In a further experimental series avian-sarcoma-virus-induced
dog brain tumors were used as a model for interstitial irradiation of neoplastic tissue (OSTERTAG et al., 1984). These
avian-sarcoma-virus induced dog brain tumors can serve as a
primary model for human brain tumors, since these tumors are
autochthonous. Their blood supply and growth are characteristic of a primary brain tumor. The features of these
tumors closely resemble those of human anaplastic astrocytomas. The intratumoral placement of iodine-125 seeds in
anaplastic gliomas produced sharply defined calcifying
necrosis with unaffected vital tumor tissue outside the
necrosis. The calcified necrosis was complete after 90
days when the transitional zone was no longer detectable.
When compared with the necrosis in healthy brain tissue,
the volume of necrosis in neoplastic tissue was approximately 3-5 times greater. That means that there is a differential necrotizing effect of iodine-125 in normal and
neoplastic brain tissue.

CLINICAL BRACHYTHERAPY

The clinical dosimetry for permanent iodine-125-implants*
is carried out with respect of the physical and biological
properties: iodine-125 emits primarily a low energy X-ray
radiation of 27 - 35 keV. According to several investigators,
the "relative biological efficiency" (RBE) seems to be in
the range of 1.2 - 1.4 (SONDHAUS, 1981; ANDERSON and KUAN,
1981). The specific dose rate factor used for dosimetry
is 1.32 cGy per hour and mCi at 1 cm in tissue. For the
clinical situation, the calculated accumulated dose for
permanent implants ranges between 3500 and 7000 cGy. This
dose is calculated to accumulate within 90 days on the
outer radius of a tumor.
With the experimental data in mind, the dosimetry for
permanent I-125 implants is calculated on the basis of
tumor shape as indicated by CT and MR and verified
bioptically by stereotactic serial biopsies. In clinical
practice, the implantation of radioactive material is
usually carried out immediately following the stereotactic
serial biopsy, provided that the morphological diagnosis
is clear and unequivocal. Angiography of cerebral vessels,
preferably under stereotactic conditions, is a prerequisite
for each procedure (OSTERTAG et al.,1980). Implantation of
iodine-125 seeds is performed under local anaesthesia
using the Riechert stereotactic system**. Brachytherapy is
routinely used as a primary treatment for low grade gliomas
after biopsy. Occasionally it is also used to irradiate
residual tumors after incomplete surgical removal, and it is
used as a combination of external beam radiation and local
radiotherapy for high grade gliomas.

---

* supplied by 3M Comp., Medical Products Div., St. Paul,
   Minnesota, USA.

** Riechert stereotactic system manufactured by F.L. Fischer,
   7800 Freiburg, West-Germany.

RESULTS

So far, 34 patients have been treated with permanent
iodine-125 implants. All of the patients presented with
progressive neurological deficits or had evidence of
CT-controlled tumor growth or both. The majority were
astrocytic tumors (23 cases) or mixed oligo-astrocytomas
(8 cases), which were located in the thalamus-basal ganglia
or in the temporal and frontal lobes (Tab. 1-2).

Brachytherapy: Localization of Tumors

Tumorsite	No. Cases	
Basal Ganglia-Thalamus	11	
Hypothalamus	2	
Temporal Lobe - Insula	12	Tab. 1
Frontal Lobe	5	
Midbrain - Pons	3	
Pituitary	1	
Total	34	

Brachytherapy: Diagnoses of Tumors

Tumortype (WHO)	No. Cases	
Astrocytoma I	6	
Astrocytoma II	12	
Oligo-Astrocytoma II	8	Tab. 2
Anaplastic Astrocytoma III	5	
PNET	2	
Pituitary Adenoma	1	
Total	34	

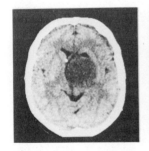 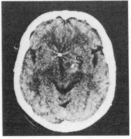

Fig.1: Stereotactic brachytherapy for a basal ganglia
astrocytoma. CT (left) demonstrates a delineated pilocytic astrocytoma (WHO I) in the left basal ganglia
of a 20 year-old female. Following a shunting procedure (white dot in right frontal horn) an iodine-125
seed (S) (activity 12.6 mCi) was implanted into the
center of the tumor. The seed delivered a calculated
dose of 6000 cGy on the outer diameter (36 mm) of the
tumor. A CT control (right) one year later revealed a
shrinkage of the tumor with a ring-like mineralization
around the implanted seed. The patient is presently
symptom-free.

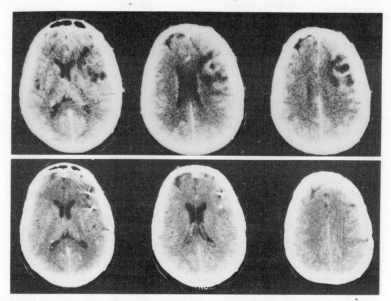

Fig.2: Stereotactic brachytherapy for a frontal astrocytoma. CT (upper) demonstrates a poorly delineated
fibrillary astrocytoma (WHO II) in the left fronto-
lateral region of a 46 year-old male. A proceeding
craniotomy had resulted in a biopsy. Two iodine-125
seeds (S) with a total activity of 10 mCi were implanted which delivered a calculated dose of 5000
cGy within a diameter of 25 mm. Distance between the
seeds was 25 mm. In a CT control eight months later
(lower) the mass effect and the edema had disappeared.
The patient is presently doing well and without a
neurological deficit.

The calculated accumulated doses ranged between 2000 cGy for
a pontine astrocytoma and 7000 cGy for a temporal lobe tumor
(mean 5500 cGy). The radius of irradiated tumors varied from
8 mm to 20 mm (mean 15.5 mm). The implants produced favorable
responses resulting in stabi- lization (14 patients) or
improvement of neurological symptoms (13 patients), which was
paralleled by a CT controlled reduction in tumor mass (Fig.
1-2). Four patients with anaplastic astrocytomas (WHO III)
and two patients with extended oligo-astrocytomas (WHO II)
received additional external beam radiotherapy with doses up
to 4000 cGy. In three patients with anaplastic astrocytomas,
the combined irradiation did not halt clinical deterioration.
These patients died within 3,4, and 6 months, respectively.
Two patients received brachytherapy for recurrent primitive
neuroectodermal tumors (PNET) of the pineal region after
previous external beam radiotherapy. Both have responded well
so far (observation times 2 months and 1 year, respectively)
There have been no complications or death related to the
operative procedure of implanting seeds.

DISCUSSION

The clinical data of this new series are considered premature and data on survival cannot be interpreted at this early
time. The larger Freiburg series, which now comprises more
than 500 cases, quotes 5 year survival rates of 54 % for
pilocytic astrocytomas, 45 % for astrocytomas grade II (WHO),
and 4 % for anaplastic astrocytomas. The survival rate for
oligodendrogliomas is 34 % after 5 years. These figures
represent, of course, very inhomogenous groups with respect
to tumor location, tumorsize, patient age and neurological
status (MUNDINGER et al., 1979; OSTERTAG et al., 1981).
Combined interstitial and external radiotherapy was mainly
developed by the Paris group with SZIKLA (1981, 1984). They
used both removable high activity sources for local
irradiation of the tumor volume and external radiation for
the greater target volume, which covers a wider area. That
allows the application of more moderate doses compared with
external beam radiotherapy alone.

Survival data published by the Paris group (SZIKLA et al.,
1984) show a 78 % survival for gliomas grade I, 69 % for
gliomas grade II, 55 % for gliomas grade III, and 19 % of
gliomas grade IV. It is understood, however, that these
groupings follow a different classification scheme and are
represent different treatment modalities. ROUGIER et al.
(1984) quote a 50 % survival rate after 5 years for
anaplastic gliomas treated with combined temporary
interstitial and external beam radiotherapy. GUTIN et al.,
1984, KELLY et al., 1978 also report favorable survival of
patients with malignant gliomas. To date, however, no
survival rates are available.

Brachytherapy with low dose rate permanent implants is not
without hazards. Complications result mainly from over-
dosage, i.e. neurological deterioration can result from
secondary effects of vasogenic edema or direct radiation
damage of functionally critical structures (KIESSLING et al.,
1984). Unwanted side effects can be avoided with careful
dosimetry. Nausea, vomiting, and somnolence syndrome,
however, commonly seen after external cranial irradiation,
are not observed after interstitial radiotherapy.

To compare interstitial radiotherapy with conventional
fractionated beam therapy is a difficult undertaking.
Prospective controlled trials on low grade gliomas have yet
to be carried out. Clinical results of both external beam
radiotherapy and interstitial radiotherapy have been based on
studies of populations of patients grouped by tumor name
only, regardless of the origin of the tumor, the age of the
patient, the clinical presentation and course, and without a
commonly accepted classification scheme. The only way to
obtain more conclusive figures is through a multicenter,
multimodality treatment study. Various centers in Europe are
currently preparing to set up such a study.

In summary, brachytherapy with I-125 permanent implants
is recommended for slowly proliferating, differentiated,
non-resectable tumors in functionally critical areas.
It enables the surgeon to achieve a radiosurgical tumor
removal while carefully avoiding radiation damage to the
normal surrounding brain, which is of particular importance in long-term survivers. Brachytherapy with iodine-125
permanent implants is effective for local tumor control,
and is, at the same time, the least traumatic treatment
when carefully applied. External beam radiation therapy
alone should not be given unless microscopic examination
of tumor tissue reveals evidence of anaplastic changes
and infiltrative growth. Combined interstitial and external
beam radiotherapy, which allows the application of more
moderate doses, compared with external beam radiotherapy
alone, has proved useful for the treatment of localized
anaplastic gliomas.

Acknowledgements:

This work is supported in part by the Deutsche
Forschungsgemeinschaft (Os 58/2-1) and the Deutsche
Krebshilfe e.V. (M 37/84/OS 1).

References

Anderson L.L., H.M. Kuan, I.Y. Ding (1981). In: Modern
   Interstitial and Intracavitary Radiation Cancer
   Management, F.W. George (ed.), Masson, New York.
Blasberg R.G., J.D. Fenstermacher, C.S. Patlak (1983).
   J. Cereb. Blood Flow Metab. 3, 8-32.
Burger P.C., M.S. Mahaley, L. Dudka, F.S. Vogel (1979).
   Cancer 44, 1256-1272.
Caveness W.F. (1980). In: Radiation Damage to the
   Nervous System, H.A. Gilbert and A.R. Kagan (eds.),
   Raven Press, New York.
Groothuis D.R., D.C. Wright, Ch.B. Ostertag (1985),
   in press.
Gutin P.H., T.L. Phililips, W.M. Wara, S.A. Leibel,
   Y. Hosobuchi, V.A. Levin, K.A. Weaver, S. Lamb (1984).
   J. Neurosurg. 60, 61-68.

Hoshino T., M. Barker, Ch.B. Wilson, E.B. Boldrey,
    D. Fewer (1972). J. Neurosurg. 37, 15-25.
Hoshino T. (1984). J. Neurosurg. 61, 895-900.
Janzer R.C., P. Kleihues, Ch.B. Ostertag (1985).
    Acta Neuropathol., in press.
Kelly P.J., M.H. Olson, A.E. Wright (1978).
    Surg. Neurol. 18, 349-354.
Kiessling M., P. Kleihues, E. Gassega, F. Mundinger,
    Ch. B. Ostertag, K. Weigel (1984). Acta Neurochir.,
    Suppl. 33, 281-289.
Kuhlendahl H., H. Miltz, R. Wüllenweber (1973). Acta
    Neurochir. 29, 151-162.
Laws E.R., W.F. Taylor, M.B. Clifton, H. Okazaki H
    (1984). J. Neurosurg. 61, 665-673.
Mundinger F., B. Busam, W. Birg, J. Schildge (1979).
    In: Stereotactic Cerebral Irradiation, INSERM Symposium
    No.12, G. Szikla (ed.), Elsevier/North Holland Bio-
    medical Press, Amsterdam.
Ostertag Ch.B., H.D. Mennel, M. Kiessling (1980).
    Surg. Neurol. 14, 275-283.
Ostertag Ch.B., F. Mundinger, K. Weigel (1981).
    Med. et Hyg. 39, 1944-2008.
Ostertag Ch.B., K.A. Hossmann, W. v.d.Kerckhoff (1982).
    Nucl.-Med. 21, 99-104.
Ostertag Ch.B., K. Weigel, P. Warnke, G. Lombeck,
    P. Kleihues (1983). Neurosurgery 13, 523-528.
Ostertag Ch.B., D. Groothuis, P. Kleihues (1984).
    Acta Neurochir., Suppl. 33, 271-280.
Ostertag Ch.B., P. Warnke, P. Kleihues, D. Bigner
    (1984). Neurol. Res. 6, 176-180.
Rougier A., J. Pigneux, F. Cohadon (1984). Acta
    Neurochir., Suppl. 33, 345-353.
Scanlon P.W., W.F. Taylor (1979). Neurosurgery 5,
    301-308.
Schiffer D., M.T. Giordana, P. Paoletti, R. Soffietti,
    L. Tarenzi (1980). Acta Neurochir. 53, 205-216.
Schiffer D., M.T. Giordana, R. Soffietti, L. Tarenzi,
    R. Milani, E. Vasario, P. Paoletti (1981). Acta
    Neurochir. 58, 37-58.
Sondhaus C.A. (1981). In: Modern Interstitial and Intra-
    cavitary Radiation Cancer Management, F.W. George (ed.),
    Masson, New York.
Szikla G., O. Betti, L. Szenthe, M. Schlienger (1981).
    Neurochirurgie 27, 295-298.
Szikla G., M. Schlienger, S. Blond, C. Daumas-Duport,
    O. Missir, S. Miyahara, A. Musolino, C. Schaub (1984).
    Acta Neurochir., Suppl. 33, 355-362.
Zeman W. (1968). In: Pathology of the Nervous System,
    J. Minckler (ed.), pp. 864-939, McGraw-Hill, New York.

The Treatment of Low-grade Malignant Brain Tumors with Stereotactic Brachytherapy

F. Frank, A. P. Fabrizi, R. Frank-Ricci
and G. Gaist

Division of Neurosurgery, Bellaria Hospital, Bologna, Italy

ABSTRACT

In 5 years, 37 patients were treated with stereotactic I^{125} implants for the treatment of low malignant tumors considered inoperable due to their deep seated and/or highly functional cerebral locations. Our experience shows that the results obtained were positive in a high percentage of the cases, with a survival rate of 78.4%, and moreover the quality of life in these patients was excellent in 86.2%, with complete social reinsertment. The follow-up (6 months-5 years) shows that the neoplasms which best respond to brachytherapy are homogenous, well-defined oligodendrogliomas and astrocytomas (grade II). The tumors that respond poorly to treatment with I^{125} are calcified neoplasms and chiasmatic gliomas.

KEYWORDS

Serial stereotactic biopsies; radioisotopic implantations; iodine 125; low-grade malignant neoplasms; social reinsertment.

INTRODUCTION

Low-grade cerebral neoplasms in deep seated areas with difficult or impossible surgical approaches, or in highly functional regions have posed difficult therapeutic problems. The elevated morbidity concerning direct surgical approaches and scarse results obtained with traditional radiotherapy have favored the use of isotopic implantations, by means of stereotaxy in the treatment of these tumors. The neoplasms,which best respond to stereotactic brachytherapy, must be of low grade and must not exceed 4.5 cm. in maximum diameter.

MATERIALS AND METHOD

From 1980 to 1984 low energy radioisotopic implants, after serial
biopsies, have been performed in 37 patients with inoperable neoplasms, located in various sites and of different histological types. Table 1 presents the site and histological nature of the treated tumors. Table 2 presents a 6 month to 5 year follow-up of the
patients, whom are still alive after the implant (8 patients(27.4%)
have died prior to the follow-up within 8-36 months from the implant). This table shows of the 29 patients whom are still alive,
20 (69%) are in good health with disappearance or reduction of the
neoplasm at CT controls; while of the remaining 9 patients, 5
(17.2%) presented with unmodified neoplasms at radiological control
and 4 patients (13.8%) worsened clinically due to the onset of peritumoral demielinization.
The implants were performed by means of stereotaxy, after reconstruction of CT images on peroperative skull Xrays. All the implants,
with the exception of children, were executed under local anesthe-
sia, and after definitive histological diagnoses (H&E preparations).
The maximum diameter of the lesions was less than 4.5 cm. in diameter. The Riechert Stereotactic frame was used for the stereotaxic interventions. (Fischer, Inc., Frieburg, I.Br., Germany.)
The isotope implanted was Iodine ^{125}, a low energy radiation emit-
ter. This radioisotope was chosen for the following characteristics:
    1)half-life of 60.2 days-a relatively short period to evaluate
       the outcome of the treatment.
    2)short radius of maximum activity (2.5 cm. from the source)-
       neither special protective measures, nor isolation of the
       patients are necessary.
The patients after a few days from the permanent implant are sent
home and reinserted into their daily routine.

DISCUSSION

The use of radioisotopes in the treatment of inoperable brain tumors is not a novelty. This method was first employed in France in
the early '60s by the Paris school (Tallairach)[9]. After a period
of abandonment, with the arrival of more precise neuroradiological
instruments (CT scanner) and the basis of more precise spatial vo-
lumeteric tumoral calculation, there was a resprouting of stereotactic brachytherapy[3,4,5,6]. There was also a shift in the isotopes
used; and two major currents arose, an american[1,2]and european[3,7,8]
trend for the treatment of brain tumors with interstitial radiotherapy. While the american school uses high energy radioisotopes with
an "after-loading" technique in the treatment of malignant gliomas;
the european objective is the treatment of low malignant gliomas,
using permanent low energy isotope implants. The characteristics
of the isotope employed in our work (I^{125}) was previously discussed. I^{125} has a short half-life, therefore it is possible to evaluate the efficacy of the treatment in 3-4 months. It should also be
pointed out that an immediate response to the treatment of the neo-

plasms (from a neuroradiological viewpoint) does not imply a complete cure of the patient. The patient must be followed by periodic control CT examinations to see eventual recurrences or the appearance of radionecrosis. The tumoral recurrence can not be fore-
seen, and maybe due to numerous factors; among these:isotope hypo-
dosage. The radionecrosis may appear after a period of latency,
starting at one year and becoming well evident at 18 months. This
manifestation is more worrisome of subcortical tumors, and less
frequent in deep seated neoplasms. This may depend on the fact that
subcortical tumors are more spread out, and may necessitate a greater isotopic charge than small, circumscribed, deep seated lesions. When radionecrosis does appear in subcortical tumors, there
is an intense surrounding edemegenous reaction, that may involve
an entire hemisphere (fig.1). Some Aa. believe (Ostertag)6 that this
reaction is caused by vasogenic edema, slowly reversible with cor-
ticosteroid therapy. We believe that this abnormal response is due
to demielinization of the peritumoral white matter; and this effect
does not subside in time. Steroid therapy is effective in reducing
swelling and the mass effect, however it is impotent towards the
perifocal demielinizing isotope induced reaction.
In deep seated tumors radionecrosis may assume a cystic aspect
(fig. 2). Once the cyst is aspirated by means of stereotaxy, the
clinical and radiological aspects maybe completely resolved. The
cystic and edemegenous responses appear in a small percentage of
the patients treated, the majority respond well to the brachytherapy with progressive reduction and eventual disappearance of the
neoplasm (fig. 3&4). At times there maybe an arrest in the reduction of the mass; however this does not imply that the isotope
was ineffective, but moreover the formation of a sclerotic and cal-
cific intra- and perineoplastic barrier (Ostertag)6 Only an arrest
of the clinical symptoms and CT controls in time may confirm this
hypothesis, and a re-biopsy may prove it.
In our series of patients treated with I^{125} we have observed a relatively low morbidity (13.8%); while the majority have resumed
their work and social activities (86.2%). The patients,who deceased
in time (21.6%), led normal lives after the implant; and died either due to a histological grading error or because of a malignant
transformation of their neoplasm. The problem of a histopathological grading error must be taken into account, because the stereotactic biopsy, although performed in a serial fashion, does not
examine the entire tumoral mass. The high malignant transformation
of the neoplasm may occur without any treatment; however in some
cases the anaplastic transformation maybe hypothetically due to the
stimulating action of the implanted isotope.

CONCLUSIONS

The Aa!s 5 year experience with stereotactically implanted isotopes
in the treatment of low malignant brain tumors presents the following conclusions:
    I)The procedure is valid because it permits prolonged survival
    with complete social reinsertment.

II)There is a low mortality rate, although the mortality pends
on a histopathological grading error.
III)The Aa. believe that the isotope dosage problems maybe overcome by greater volumetric definition provided by nuclear
magnetic resonance (NMR).

Table 1: Site and histological nature of the neoplasms treated
with permanent I^{125} implants.
(1980-1984)

HISTOLOGICAL TYPES		TUMORAL SITES	
Subependymomas	2	Frontal lobe	9
Pineocytomas	2	Parietal lobe	2
Craniopharyngiomas	3	Temporal lobe	2
Oligodendroglioma	1	Suprasellare reg.	6
Astrocytomas (Gr.II)	27	Pineal region	7
Ependymoma	1	third ventricle	3
Pituitary adenoma	1	Basal ganglia	5
		Brainstem	3
Total	37		37

Table 2: Follow-up of the patients that underwent I^{125} implants
(6 months-5 years)

CLINICAL-RADIOLOGICAL
RESULTS

	Pats.		
Good	20	Complete Social	
Fair	5	Reinsertment	(86.2%)
Unsatisfactory	4	Physical disability	(13.8%)
Total	29		

* 8 out of 37 patients died within 8-36 months from the
implant prior to the follow-up.

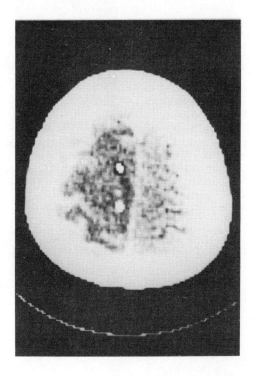

Fig.1. 18 y/o female with a left frontal subcorti-
        cal grade II astrocytoma. CT image 3 years
        after the implant shows no neoplasm, but an
        enormous left hemispheric demielinization.
        (2 grains of I125 implanted)

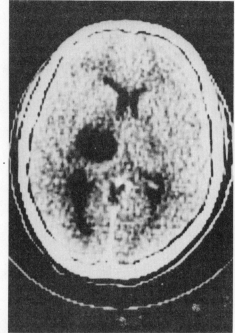

Fig.2.   16 y/o male with a
         left thalamic astro-
         cytoma.

A) After 2 years from
   the implant, the
   appearance of a col-
   liquated necrotic
   cyst.

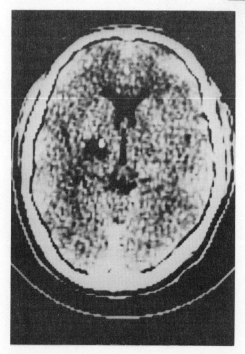

B) Result after stereo-
   tactic aspiration of
   the cystic content.

(1 grain of I^{125})

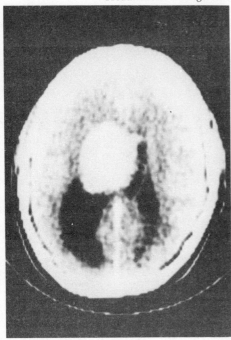

Fig.3. 20 y/o female with a
        left deep frontal oli-
        dendroglioma.

A) Prior to the implant.

B) 4 years after the im-
   plantation.

   (2 grains of I^{125})

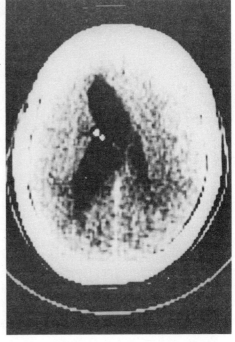

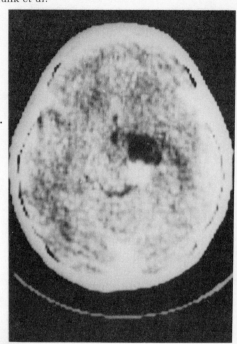

Fig.4. 7 y/o girl with a
right deep temporal
astrocytoma; in part
solid, in part cystic.

A)CT image prior to
the implant.

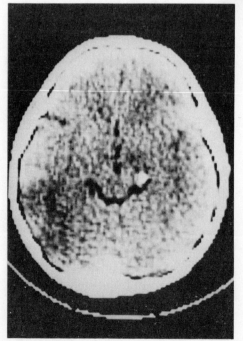

B) 5 years after the implant;
total radiological disap-
pearance of the tumor.

(1 grain of I125)

REFERENCES

1. Gutin,P.H., Phillips,T.L., Hosobuchi,Y., Wara,W.M., MacKay,A.R.,
   Weaver,K.A., Lamb,S., Hurst,S. Permanent and removable implants
   for the brachytherapy of brain tumors. Int.J.Radiat.Oncol.Biol.
   Phys. 1981;21:1371-81.

2. Lundsford,D. Personal communication: "Brachytherapy in malignant
   gliomas". From the World Stereotaxic Meeting, held in Toronto,
   Canada, 4-7 July, 1985.

3. Mundinger,F. The treatment of brain tumors with interstitially
   applied radioisotopes. In: Yen Wang and Paoletti,F., eds. Ra-
   dionucleotide applications in neurology and neurosurgery.
   Springfield,Ill.: Charles C. Thomas, 1970: 199-265.

4. Mundinger,F. Implantation of Radioisotopes (Curie-Therapy).
   In: Stereotaxy of the human brain, eds. Georges Schaltenbrand
   and A. Earl Walker. Stuttgart;New York: Georg Thieme Verlag,
   1982:410-435.

5. Ostertag,C.B., Mennel,H.D., Kiessling,M. Stereotactic biopsy of
   brain tumors. Surg. Neurol. 1980;14:275-283.

6. Ostertag,C.B. Biopsy and interstitial radiation therapy of cerebral gliomas. Ital. J. Neurol. Sci. (Suppl.2) 1983: 121-8.

7. Pecker,J., Scarabin,J.M., Brucher,J.M., Vallée,B. Démarche stéréotaxique en neurochirurgie tumorale.(Stereotactic approach to
   diagnosis and treatment of cerebral tumors.) Paris: Laboratoires
   Pierre Fabre, 1979:87-98 (In French).

8. Szikla,G., Betti,O., Szenthe,L., Schlienger,M. L'éxperience
   actuelle des irradiations stéréotaxiques dans le traitement des
   gliomas hémisphériques. Neurochirurgie (Paris) 1981;27:295-298.

9. Talairach,J., Bonis,G.,Szikla,G.,Schaub,G., Baucaud,J., Covello,
   L., Bordas-Ferrer,F. Stereotaxic implantation of radioactive isotopes in functional pituitary surgery. Techniques and results.
   In: Yen Wang and Paoletti,F., Radionuclide applications in neurology and Neurosurgery, Thomas, Springfield,Ill., 1970: 267-325.

External Stereotactic Irradiation of Human Gliomas by Linear Accelerator

F. Colombo*, A. Benedetti*, L. Casentini*,
F. Pozza**, R. C. Avanzo***, G. Chierego*** and
C. Marchetti***

*Department of Neurosurgery, City Hospital, Vicenza, Italy
**Department of Radiotherapy, City Hospital, Vicenza, Italy
***Service of Medical Physics, City Hosptial, Vicenza, Italy

ABSTRACT

The Authors describe the results obtained in a series of 36 patients
harboring intracranial tumors treated by an original technique of externally
focalized stereotactic irradiation allowing the administration of high doses
(2000-5000 rads) in one or two sessions.Follow up ranges from 31 to 6
months.In the Authors opinion this technique seems to be particularly
indicated in low grade gliomas,malignat radiosensible tumors,heavily
vascularized tumors and arteriovenous malformations.

INTRODUCTION

As stated by Gabor szikla in his preface to the book Stereotactic Cerebral
Irradiation "high dose focal irradiation limited to the lesion may destroy
small tumors without inflicting significant damage to adjacent brain,also in
important and vulnerable areas,provided that the irradiated volume corresponds
closely to that of the tumor.The indispensable precision of both localization
and irradiation can be obtained by stereotactic techniques only"(Szikla,1979).
This is the rationale of stereotactic irradiation,a concept by passing
the problems oftumor radiosensitivity and radionecrosis,relying only on
three dimensional resolution:a way of thinking more close to the mind of
stereotactic surgeon("Radiosurgery") than to that of the radiotherapist.
Untill now,two groups of techniques of stereotactic irradiation have been
widely investigated and employed in clinical practice:the radioisotopes
infixion techniques(Mundinger,1979)and the external beam radiosurgical
procedures(Leksell,1971,Kjellberg et al,1972),both these techniques aiming
to the destruction(radionecrosis) of the tumor volume.
The use of external beam stereotactic irradiation has not gained wide use
owing to the high cost of the radiation machines(Gamma Unit,Cyclosyncrotrone).
We have developped and introduced in clinical practice a radiosurgical
technique employing a isocentric linear accelerator(Colombo et al,1984,1985).
With this technique We have treated 47 patients affected by intracranial

tumors and arteriovenous malformations.For 36 of them We have a follow up
longer than 6 months.17 patients harbored glial tumors.This paper will
deal with them.

MATHERIAL AND METHODS

The technique employed has been described elsewhere(Colombo et al,1984,1985).
Basically,it can be defined as a multiple isocentric arc irradiations with
small fields centered in the stereotactic target.
After the fixation of the patient's head to the stereotactic helmet,the
tumor volume is defined in three dimensional space by standard
neuroradiological study(CT scan,Angiography) and verified by stereotactic
biopsy.In a following step the helmet is fixed to the treatment couch
of our Varian Clinac 4 MV linear accelerator by a particular adaptor.
The target is made to coincide with the linear accelerator isocenter.
A first irradiation is undertaken on a 100°-140° arc.The treatment couch
is then rotated of 10°-20° degreees around a vertical axis passing throgh
the target and the arc irradiations are repeated on 5-17 planes distributed
on a 160° cylindrical sector.The dose gradient obtained is very steep.
Field dimensions are selected for having the 80% isodose(where the dose
gradient is steeper)coinciding with the tumor volume.
With this technique large doses can be delivered in one or two sessions.

RESULTS

Our series consists. of 36 patients with a follow-up ranging from 31 to 6
months.Patients with follow-up shorter than six months(11 other raising the
total number to 47) are not considered here.
All patients (except AVMs) have had a positive histological verification
before radiosurgery(30 by multiple stereotactic biopsy sampling and 3 by
craniotomy mass reduction procedures).
All patients were deemed not suitable to "classical" neurosurgical procedures.
At the beginning of our trial We were very often confronted with patients
that were desesperately hill,sometimes with serious general problems that
complicated the neurological disease.I confess that some of the desolate
cases were treated only "ut aliquid fecisse videatur"(one patient with
a germinoma,two cases with anaplastic gliomas,one case with a glioblastoma
and one case with metastasis).These patients should be refuses.
We strongly fought to have the autopsy verification in patients that succumbed.
This was not possible in patients died at home or at the hospital of
referral,sometimes many undredth of kilometers from Vicenza.
Three patients died in our hospital and these were verified.Three patients
were operated on;all in our department and the specimen underwent a thoroughly
histological verification.One patient underwent stereotactic biopsy after
radiosurgery.

Low grade atsrocitomas: clinical results can be defined good also if the
follow up is short.All patients were treated with two shots of 800-2500
rads,according to the volume,the location of the tumor and the age of
of the patient.
A result that can be considered usual is shown by patient number 3.

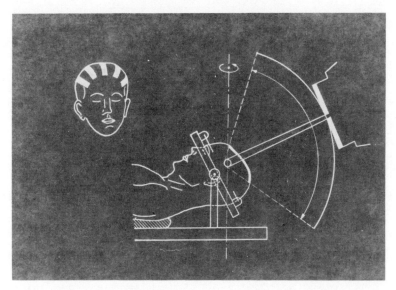

FIG.1:linear accelerator radiosurgery principle:to multiply concentric arc
irradiations by rotating the patient around a vertical axis passing through
the target

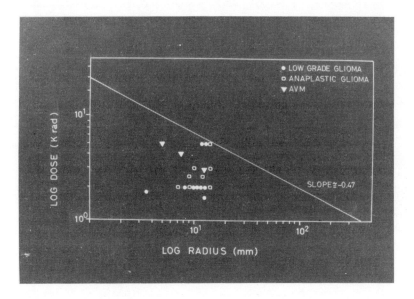

FIG.2:diagram log dose vs log radius of treated lesions

This patient,a 9 years old boy was affected by a large thalamic pylocytic
astrocytoma.With two sessions of only 800 rads We were able to follow the
complete evolution of the modifications induced by radiosurgical treatment.
One month after treatment the lesion (unenhanced preoperatively)took
massively the contrast.Two months after treatment at CT scan appeared a
typical"ring feature" that slowly increased in size for approximatively
2 months. The patient had some minor problems such as morning headache
which subsided to Dexametazone treatment (16 mg die for 2 weeks).
From the sixth month,the clinical and neuroradiological situation went on
improving.Now the clinical picture is completetly normal and the CT shows
an almost complete shrinkage of the lesion.
Similar very good results were obtained in 5 out of 9 patients.Two patients
(13 months follow-up) are unchanged.

anaplastic gliomas behave more aggressively.Out of 7 patients,2 died of their
disease at 6 and 9 months(no autopsy performed).One case was operated 4
months after irradiation.One patient was lost in the follow-up 12 months
after radiosurgery.Two patients (affected by thalamic anaplastic astrocytomas)
are in good conditions after 27 and 11 months with a complete shrinkage
of the lesion.One of these two patient,after two stereotactic boost of
1100 rads in the solid part,required the treatment of the cystic part of her
right thalamic anaplastic astrocytoma with Colloidal Rhenium.This treatment
was done in an other Institute,3 moths after radiosurgery.During this
procedure bioptic sampling of the solid part was repeated.This component
was found to be almost completely necrotic.The original mass lesion
seems to be now completely shrinked(21 months).
Two patients went on worsening despite radiosurgery.Both of them harbored
large lesions(3 and 3.5 cm) with important cystic or necrotic components.
Beside this,the lesions had a very irragular three dimensional configuration,
hard to cover with a spherical isodose.One of these patient was operated
on for increasing intracranial pressure.Pathological specimen was almost
superimposable to the bioptic specimen taken before radiosurgery.

oligodendrogliomas;two patients were treated with two shots of 1000 rads.
Clinical and CT picture are unchanged at 18 and 12 months.

ependymomas.Two thalamic lesions were classified as ependymoma.One patient
had a very large tumor,that displayed at histological examination many
features of active proliferation.Two boost of 2500 rads produced a massive
necrotization of the tumor but the mass effect remained unchanged at six months.
Aeras of hypodensity were also present in the brain surrounding the tumor
(edema?radionecrosis?).The patient died at his home 9 months after
radiosurgery.No autopsy performed.
The second patient had a small lesion,histologically benign,that was treated
with two sessions of 1100 rads.The clinical picture is now completely normal
and the lesion unrecognizable at CT (6 months follow-up).

pinealomas.One patient affected by a pineocytoma was treated with 2 X 1500 rads
The lesion (highly enhanced with contrast media before radiosurgery) showed
the appearance of a ring feature three months after radiosurgery,with a

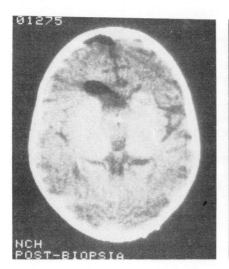 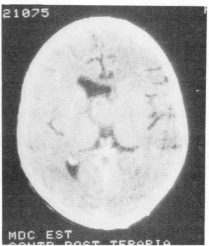

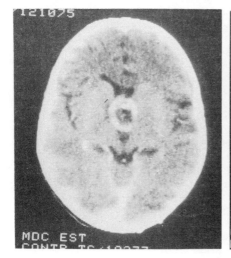 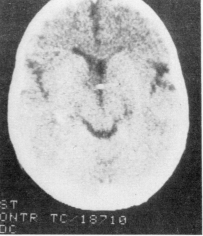

FIG.3:CT follow up of patient n° 3

limited shrinkage.The Parinaud's syndrome and the raised intracranial
pressure were definitively relived.
The patient died for chronic liver insufficency 12 months after.At autopsy,
no evidence of radionecrosis in the adjacent brain stem.The core of the
lesion was largely necrotic with hyalinosis of the vessels wall.
A young girl with a pinealoblastoma was treated with two shots of 1000 rads
combined with large fields,fractioned doses radiotherapy(3000 rads).
Complete regression of the mass was evident one month after radiosurgery.
She's recurrence free till today(31 months after).
Two patients were affected by germinomas.One of them(a young man aged 18)
harboring a intraventricular mass 35 mm in diameter was seriously hill.
He had a long standing bilateral amaurosis and hypothalamic insufficiency.
Two episodes of renal failure required dialitic treatment.Brain stem
compression entailed an impaired consciousness and tetraparesis.
He was treated with a single shot of 1000 rads.15 days after the
lesion was almost completely desappeared at CT.The patient died 32 days
after.At autopsy,no evidence of radionecrosis.The lesion,completely necrotic,
was a small reddish mass of 0.7 cm,The other patient(14 years old boy,
harboring a germinoma of the pineal gland,2.2 cm in diameter)after 1000 rads
had a resolution of the Parinaud's syndrome and a desappearance of the
lesion at CT scan after only 4 days!The treatment was completed with
3000 rads extended fields,refracted dose onthe neuraxis.After 12 months,
CT and neurological picture remain normal.

Medulloblastoma:similar treatment and similar results were obtained in
a 18 years old male affected by a large(3.5 cm) medulloblastoma infiltrating
the upper brain stem and the posterior part of the third ventricle.
With 2000 rads no mass at CT and normalization of the clinical picture
after one month.With radiotherapic complement(3000 rads) the situation is
unchanged 19 months after.

Meningioma:the unresectable part of an angioblastic meningioma infiltrating
the cavernous sinus was left in place during a craniotomy procedure performed
on a 42 years old female.This large mass(2.5 cm) caused complete cavernous
sinus syndrome with exophtalmos,chemosis,oftalmoplegia,unbearable first
division pain.6 months after surgery the patient was treated with two
sessions of 1250 rads each.The lesion gradually shrinked(complete regression
at 12 months)with marked clinical improvement(regression of exophtalmos
and pain syndrome).

Metastasis:One patient(male,aged 53)affected by a unique metastasis of a
lung epithelial carcinoma was treated with 2000 rads stereotactically
targetted in the lesion(2.5 cm) plus 3000rads large field,refracted doses.
He died 13 months after for disseminated metastatic disease 15 months
after.At autopsy,no evidence of the lesion surrounding the metallic marker
inserted in the biopsy site.The other patient(male,aged 56)died 6 months
after treatment.Autopsy was refused.

Craniopharyngiomas:a 6 years old boy affected by a intraventricular lesion
with a large solid component was treated with a single shot of 700 rads.
Cystic part was punctured and evacuated.The mass is unchanged 17 months after.

No recurrence of the cystic part.The other patient was treated with 800 raas
in the solid part.Mass effect is still present and worsening(poor result).

arteriovenous malformations:three patients with thalamic arteriovenous
malformations were treated with two sessions of 2000 rads each.A minor
hemorrhage recurred 1 month after in one of them.Clinical picture is
unchanged in all patients.Follow-up angiography is planned one year after
treatment.

PATHOLOGY

We were able to examine pathology specimens of 4 patients,two of them
harboring gliomas.One patient affected by an anaplastic astrocitoma was
operated on 4 months after for incresing intracranial pressure.Any significative
change wasn't detected.
The single patient affected by a glioblastoma was also operated on 6 months
after radiosurgery.The histological specimen showed an increased in size
necrotic area;multiple,polynucleated giant cells with signs of cytotoxicity
were also prominent.But also vital tumor tissue was still present.
The pathology of the patient affected by a pineocytoma can be of interest.
This patient,improved after radiosurgery from the neurological and CT points
of view,died 12 months after for a liver disease.At autopsy the tumor had
a ischemic central core,while the vessels were affected by massive hyalinosis
and endotelial proliferation .These vessels damages were lacking before
radiosurgery and were more preminent in that partof the tumor that received
the highest dosage(the center) and that was depicted,in the follo-up CTs,
as the hypodense central area of a ring feature.We think that similar
vessels damage could be involved in the evolution of irradiated low grade
gliomas and vascularized tumors.
The specimen of the third ventricle germinoma demonstrated a massive
hemorrhagic necrosis of the tumor,without any vital tissue remnant.Surrounding
nervous tissue showed no signs of redionecrosis.

DISCUSSION

Our clinical experience is to short to draw any definitive conclision.
Nevertheless two groups of tumors seem to respond very well to stereotactic
radiosurgery with linear accelerator.One is the group of low grade gliomas:
the tumor has to be well defined at CT,with clear cut borders;the dimensions
should by less than 3 cm in diameter.
In cases with favourable evolution,CT followup seem to parallel the modification
described as characteristic of low grade gliomas implanted with Iridium or
Iodine seeds(Ostertag et al,1979).We have now 7 patients with more than 12
months follow-up without any problem of late deterioration due to delayed
radionecrosis.7 patients out of nine has consistently improved or normalized
clinical picture.The treatment seem to be warranted.
The second group of highly responsive tumors is represented by an heterogeneous
mixage of malignant radiosensitive histotypes such as germinomas,pynealoblastomas
and medulloblastomas.In these patients a single stereotactically focalized
dose of 1000-1500 rads is able to obtain a rapid debulking in a very short time.
Here,the aim of radiosurgery is the same of the craniotomy procedure:to obtain

the reduction of the tumor bulk and related mass effect.the sterilization
of the entire neuraxis from seeding cells is beyond the limits of radiosurgery
and must be accomplished by standard,extended fields,refracted doses
radiotherapy.One other patient affected by a suprasellar germinoma confirmed
the usual trend with desappearance of a 2.5 cm mass in 6 days but he is
not included in the present series(follow-up three months).the combination
of radiosurgery with radiotherapy seems to be safe(three patients has a
follow up of 31,19 and 12 months).
Also if arteriovenous malformations are considered good candidates to
radiosurgery(Steiner et al,1974) their behaviour after linear accelerator
focalized irradiation is not ascertainable nowadays.The three AVMs treated
has a follow-up of 7 and 6 months(to short) and carotid angiography is
still an examination that can not be safely repeated to often;We plan to
study this group of patients one year after treatment.Nevertheless in one
patient CT control shoved a significant decrease in size of the AVM.
The angioblastic meningioma had a very satisfactory evolution with an
important decrease in size at six months and an almost complete desappearance
at 12 months.We do hope that this will be the trend of AVMs also.
The reasons why anaplastic gliomas and glioblastomas respond less to
radiosurgery are a matter of debate.One of these reasons can be that the
borders of the tumor are less well defined and many malignant cells can
be well beyond the borders of the therapeutic isodose(Daumas Duport et al,1982)
But an important factor mus be also the time the therapeutic effect takes
to develop.Often in low grade gliomas one year is indispensable to have the
shrinkage of the lesion.This time lapse could be to long for a rapid growing
tumor.In glioblastoma vital tumor cells can be identified in necrotic and
ischemic areas and these are shielded from the ionizing radiation.
Radiosurgery increases the ischemic volume and,at the employed doses,could
be not able to kill viable cells included in it.
With regard to the possible fisopathologic factors leading to the therapeutic
effect these seem to be more strictly related to the total amount of the
dose than to radiation time schedule or fractionation.This fact is in
agreement with an aspecific damage induced by the dose focalized inside the
target volume.On the other side,owing to the well known low proliferating
fraction of low grade gliomas(Hoshino,1984) a cycling cells specific agent
must be rejected.
The time lapse from the radiosurgical treatment to the actual shrinkage of
the tumor is more critical in slow growing tumors:in most of the patients
the therapeutic effect took 9-12 months to be completed.In the first 6 months
a temporary increase of the mass effect,seldom requiring major therapeutic
maneuvers,should be expected.
But the main problem to be solved is the choice of the amount of dose to be
delivered.Radiosurgical experience at the Karolinska(employing much higher
doses) is not superimposable.Our collimator openings are different(usually
larger).Our dose gradient for small fields seems to be steeper of that of
the Gamma Unit but for large fields the trend is reversed.On the other side
the Kjellberg diagram radius vs dose for radiosurgical procedures is based
on few cases and has a large range of unreliability(Kjellberg,1979).
The decision on the dose is still hard stuff.
Evaluating our experience We can find some clues but few certainities.
Two irradiations of only 800 rads with a 3 X3 cm field was sufficent to
shrink a low grade gliomas.But also two shots of 2500 rads each with a

a 3 X 3 cm field in five arcs were well tolerated.The only patient with suspected problems of radionecrosis received two shots of 2500 rads with a field 4 X 4 cm.Obviously the lowest efficent dose must be actively searched. Standard radiotherapy relies upon a selective sensitivity of the proliferating tomur cells while radiosurgery effect depends only on the dose delivered irrespectively to the pathology of the target.As suggested by Steiner(1984) and Barcia Salorio(1984) radiosurgery therapeutic effect could be mediated by a tumor vessels occlusion(and this fact seems supported by our scanty post radiosurgery pathological evidence). In the other hand the dramatic reduction and necrotization of higgly malignant tumors induced by a single dose in a very short time span(a costant feature of germinomas and "small cells" malignant tumors) remains still unexplained.

REFERENCES
Barcia Salorio J.L.,M.Cerda,G.Hernandez,V.Border,J.Beraha,C.Calabuig, J.Broseta(1984)Acta Neurochir. suppl.33,317-322
Colombo F.,A.Benedetti,L.Casentini,F.Pozza(1984) Min.Med 75,1327-1331
Colombo F.,A.Benedetti,F.Pozza,R.C.Avanzo,C.Marchetti,G.Chierego,A.Zanardo (1985) Neurosurgery 16,154-160
Colombo F.:Radiosurgery with linear accelerator:technical note.Proceedings First International Symposium on Advanced Technology in Neurosurgery, Milan,Italy
Daumas Duport C.,V.Monsaingeon,L.Szenthe,G.Szikla (1982) Appl.Neurophysiol.45, 431-437
Hoshino T.(1984) J.Neurosurg 61,895-901
Kjellberg R.N.,N.C.Nguyen,B.Kliman(1972) Neurochirugie 18,235-274
Kjellberg R.N.(1979) Isoeffective dose parameters for brain necrosis in relation to radiosurgical dosimetry,Proceedings of the INSERM Symposium no 12,Paris,France
Leksell L.(1971) Stereotaxy and radiosurgery:an operative system,Thomas, Springfield,Illinois
Mundinger F.(1979) Rationale and Methods of interstitial Ir 192 brachycurie therapy and Ir 192 and I 125 protracted long term irradiation,Proceedings of the INSERM Symposium no 12,Paris,France
Ostertag C.,K.Weigel,W.Birg(1979) CT changes after long term interstitial irradiation,Proceedings of the INSERM Symposium no 12,Paris,France
Steiner L.,L.Leksell,D.Forster,T.Greitz,O.Backlund(1974) Acta Neurochir. suppl.21,195-210
Steiner L.(1982) Radiosurgery in arteriovenous malformations of the brain in Textbook of cerebrovascular surgery,Springer,Berlin
Szikla G.(1979) Stereotactic Cerebral Irradiations,Elsevier,Amsterdam, Holland

Pathology of Gliomas and Normal Nervous Tissue Following Radiotherapy

M. T. Giordana

The 2nd Neurological Clinic, University of Turin, Italy

ABSTRACT

Morphological changes produced by radiotherapy in malignant gliomas are described. In many cases, changes can be observed also in the surrounding normal nervous tissue, both as peritumoral regressive areas and as typical radionecrosis.

KEYWORDS

Radiotherapy; gliomas; normal nervous tissue; pathology.

The goal of therapeutic irradiation is to achieve selective death of tumor cells. Biologically, ionizing radiation interacts ultimately with cellular DNA which may be damaged directly or, more frequently, indirectly.

The direct mechanism is typical of high LET radiations (fast neutrons, charged heavy particles). Low LET radiations (X and gamma rays) act through an indirect mechanism: their interaction with the molecules of water produces free radicals, which extract hydrogen atoms from DNA molecules. An adequate concentration of oxygen enhances the damage; hypoxia favors the endogenous protective agents which repair the damaged DNA.

Immediate death occurs in peculiarly sensitive cells only, which undergo intermitotic death. Intermitotic death, or interphase death, is the only way from which non-proliferating cells, for example neurons, can die. However, doses much higher than those currently employed in therapy are required.

Cell death results largely from mitotic or reproductive death, that is the inability of damaged cells to continually reproduce. It affects proliferating elements and is seen during the first or subsequent attempts of division, reducing the potentiality for tumor growth or metastasis. Slowly proliferating cells, such as normal endothelial and glial cells, undergo mitotic death after a very long latency.

After irradiation exposure in cultures there is exponential decline in cell survival. Tipically, a shoulder in the survival curve represents the ability of irradiated cells to accumulate and repair sublethal damage. The rate of expotential cell destruction is a measure of the true radiosensitivity of the irradiated cell population. The variability in response to irradiation seems to depend mostly on factors that affect the shoulder region of the survival curve, that is the repair capabilities.

The oxygen concentration and the position of the cell in the mitotic cycle are the factors that mostly influence the radiosensitivity. Hypoxic cells require a higher radiation dose than normally oxygenated cells to achieve the same degree of cell kill. This is due to the repair mechanisms which are favoured by hypoxia. The relatively radioresistant hypoxic cells can be responsible for tumor regrowth after irradiation.

Cells in M and S phases of the cycle have the highest sensitivity to irradiation and this is the basis of the terapeutic ratio of irradiation of cerebral tumors.

Dose fractionation, treatment under hyperbaric oxygen and chemical hypoxic cell sensitizers partly reduce the effect of hypoxic cells on tumor survival. Moreover, fractionated treatment permits repair of damage in normal cells and affects more tumor cells in the most sensitive cycle position (Soffietti et al.1984).

Malignant gliomas are non-homogeneous tumors. Radiation generates histological alterations in brain tumors which are non-specific and hardly distinguishable from those spontaneously occurring. The most reliable way to detect them is to study their frequency in relation to clinico-radiotherapeutic parameters.

In our experience, the comparison between small surgical biopsies and autopsy material is not a reliable tool to identifying morphological variations due to therapy. Only large series of brains, examined by means of the whole mount preparation, entitle to state statistical relationships between changes such as mitoses, necroses, proliferative zone, montrous cells, proliferation and degeneration of vessel walls, edema, macrophage-filled areas, and treatment modalities such as total survival, radiation dose, time interval between radiation and histological examination, chemotherapy (Burger et al. 1979; Schiffer et al.1980).

The time interval between radiation and histological examination and the total radiation dose are very important factors in the evaluation of the effects of radiotherapy.

Until 1500 rads, no changes can be found; with higher doses, immediate and late damages are observed. The former include: enlargement of the central necrosis, increased number of macrophage areas, stop of mitoses in parenchymal and endothelial cells, appearance of vessel degenerations (Fig.1) and bizarre nuclei (Fig.2). All these changes indicate a regression of the tumor.

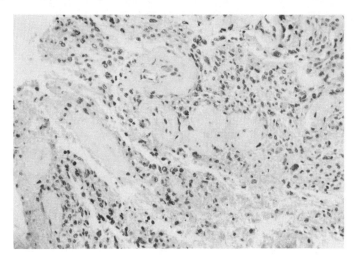

Fig.1 - Hyaline degeneration of vessel walls. H.E., 200 x.

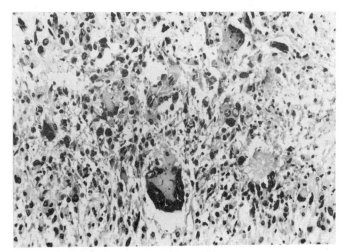

Fig.2 - Nuclear monstrosities. H.E., 400 x.

However, as it is known, malignant gliomas, even though severely damaged by irradiation and temporarely shrinked, continue to grow until the patient's death. Six months after 6000 rads, repopulation phenomena are clearly evident together with late damages: reappearance of mitoses and circumscribed necroses with pseudopalizadings, (Fig.3), reproliferation of both normal and degenerated vessels. The regrowth takes place not only in the brain surrounding the tumor,

but also in islands of viable cells surviving in the large central
necrosis (Schiffer et al.1980, 1982). Generally, it is given by
small, hyperchromatic cells (Giangaspero and Burger, 1983).

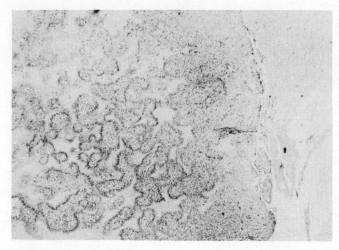

Fig.3 - Circumscribed necroses with pseudopalizadings in a regrowing
        tumor. H.E., 350 x.

The temporary clinical efficacy of radiotherapy on malignant gliomas is generally acknowledged, whereas its usefulness on low grade
astrocytomas is still a matter of discussion. Moreover, little is
known of the histological effects of radiation on these tumors,al-
so because of their long survival. Some informations about short
term effects have been obtained by studing the astrocytomatous
areas of irradiated glioblastomas (the so-called secondary glioblastomas).
The irradiated astrocytomatous areas do not greatly differ from the
typical morphological picture of astrocytoma and show no changes
referable to irradiation, provided they are not affected by chronic
edema. The low turnover of glia cells and the lacking of mitoses in
astrocytomas may account for the absence of short term effects. It
cannot be excluded that a delayed necrosis may develop through the
mechanism of mitotic death, after a long latency period (Schiffer
et al.1984).
On the contrary, morphological changes are quite evident in astrocytomas after interstitial irradiation: necrosis of tumor tissue
close to the source and less striking lesions in perifocal areas
(Kiessling et al.1983). The theoretical advantage of continuous
low dose rate irradiation is the enhancement of the therapeutic ratio, thanks to differences in repair efficiency, reoxygenation, re-
distribution through the cell cycle (Gutin and Bernstein, 1984).
The damage to the normal nervous tissue produced by irradiation of

cerebral tumors is of paramount importance. A series of changes can
be found, but only a statistical evaluation of their frequency in
relation to clinico-therapeutic parameters allows to draw conclusions on their relation with radiation. In Table 1 the changes independent of, influenced by, produced by irradiation are indicated.
The mechanism of their genesis directly or indirectly involves the
peritumoral chronic edema (Fig. 4), which occurs both spontaneously
and as a consequence of irradiation. In irradiated brains, on the
basis of dosimetric considerations, edema does not appear as entirely attributable to radiation: myelin pallor prevails in the hemisphere with the tumor, instead of being simmetrical (Schiffer et
al. 1981). Edematous peritumoral tissue results to be highly sensitive to radiation; in fact , changes produced by radiotherapy, such as
macrophage areas (Fig. 5),vessel wall degeneration (Fig. 6), necrotic areas, bizarre astrocytes (Fig. 7), are prominent in peritumoral position (Fig. 8).

TABLE 1 -   RADIOTHERAPY OF MALIGNANT GLIOMAS.

HISTOLOGICAL ALTERATIONS IN PERITUMORAL NEURAL TISSUE

1) INDEPENDENT OF RADIATION: lympho-plasmocellular infiltrates
                                cortical necroses
                                calcifications
                                peritumoral reactive astrocytes

2) INFLUENCED BY RADIATION: edema and spongiosis
                                spongio-necrosis
                                peritumoral hemorrhages
                                distant reactive astrocytes
                                scattered macrophages

3) PRODUCED BY RADIATION: bizarre astrocytes
                                vessel wall pathology
                                teleangectasias
                                peritumoral macrophage areas
                                peritumoral necroses

The major hazard of radiotherapy of brain tumors is delayed radionecrosis of normal nervous tissue. It is currently defined as a
necrosis in patients presenting clinical and radiological signs of
recurrence after radiation for brain tumors, but having little or
no persistent tumor (Mikhael, 1980).
The incidence of pathologically documented radionecroses ranges
from 2 to 5%. In our series of autoptic brains bearing radiotrea-
ted malignant gliomas, 7 cases with the histological picture of
radionecrosis were found (Fig. 9). The area of coagulative necrosis (Fig. 10) with edema, myelin and axon alterations, vessel wall
degenerations, is localized in the peritumoral white matter in 6

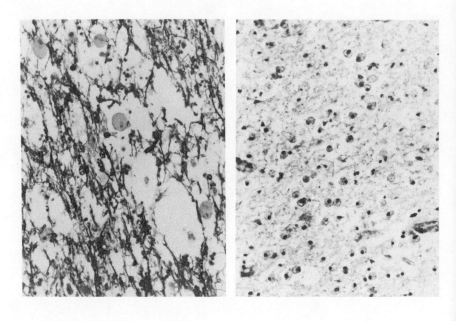

Fig.4 - Cronic edema in the
white matter. Luxol
Fast Blue B, 200 x.

Fig.5 - Macrophage area.
H.E., 200 x.

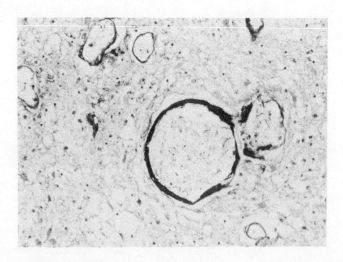

Fig.6 - Fibrinoid necrosis in the vessel walls of normal
tissue. PTAH, 400 x.

cases and in the contralateral hemisphere in one case. In three
cases, however, the tumor is large, either active quiescent; in one
case it is small but active. The analysis of isodose curve reconstruction demonstrates that the areas of radionecrosis had received the same radiation dose as the tumor, or a higher one.

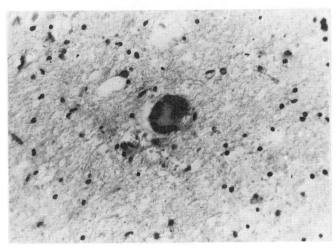

Fig.7 - Bizarre astrocyte in peritumoral tissue. H.E., 400 x.

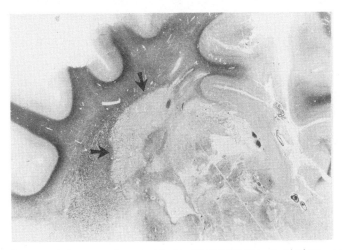

Fig.8 - Regressive area (arrows) in peritumoral position. Luxol
        Fast Blue B, 25 x.

The nervous tissue was considered to the highly radioresistant. It
is now recognized that this interpretation is false: the radiation
injury occurs, even though later; the slow turnover of
glia cells gives account for the long latency of necrotic damage.

On the other hand, a vascular pathogenesis of radionecrosis cannot be underestimated (Caveness, 1980), in line with the observation of the prominent vessel wall pathology undoubtedly related to radiation in peritumoral tissue.

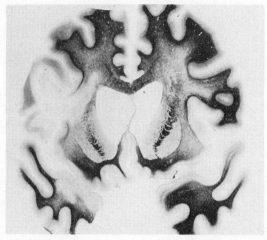

Fig.9 - Radionecrosis. Luxol Fast Blue B, 25 x.

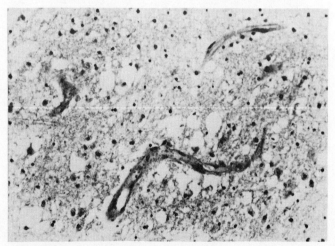

Fig.10 - Coagulative necrosis. H.E., 300 x.

ACKNOWLEDGMENT

Supported by a grant of the Italian National Research Council (C.N.R.), Special Project "Oncology", contract number 84.00796.44 and by the Italian Association for Cancer Research (A.I.R.C.).

REFERENCES
Burger, P.C., Mahaley, M.S., Dudka, L., and F.S. Vogel (1979).
Cancer 44, 1256-1272.
Caveness, W.F. (1980). In: Radiation damage the nervous system. A
delayed therapeutic hazard, Gilbert, M.A. and A.R. Kaga, eds.,
pp. 1-38, Raven Press, New York.
Giangaspero, F. and P.C. Burger (1983). Cancer 52, 2320-2333.
Gutin, P.H. and M. Bernstein (1984). Progr. exp. Tumor Res. 28,
166-182.
Kiessling, M., Kleihues,P., Mundinger, F., Ostertag, C.B., and K.
Weigel (1983). Prodeedings 6th Meeting Europ. Soc. Stereotaxic and
Functional Neurosurgery, T7, Rome, Italy.
Mikhael, M.A. (1980). In: Radiation damage to the nervous system.
A delayed therapeutic hazard. Gilbert, H.A., and R. Kagan, eds.,
pp. 59-91, Raven Press, New York.
Schiffer, D., Giordana, M.T., Paoletti, P., Soffietti, R., and L.
Tarenzi (1980). Acta Neurochir. 53, 205-216.
Schiffer, D., Giordana, M.T., Soffietti, R., Tarenzi, L., Milani,
R., Vasario, E., and P. Paoletti (1981). Acta Neurochir. 58, 37-58.
Schiffer, D., Giordana, M.T., Soffietti, R., and R. Sciolla (1982).
Acta Neuropathol. (Berl.) 58, 291-299.
Schiffer, D., Giordana, M.T., Soffietti, R., Sciolla, R., Sannazza-
ri, G.L., and E. Vasario (1984). J. Neuro-oncology 2, 167-175.
Soffietti, R., Sciolla, R., Giordana, M.T., Vasario, E., Sannazzari
G.L., and D. Schiffer (1984). Argomenti di Oncologia 5, 1-40.

Review of Epidemiological Studies on Cerebral Glioma and Presentation of a New Cooperative Study in the Veneto Region

S. Mingrino*, P. Zampieri*, R. Gallato**,
E. Di Stefano***, M. Gerosa****,
A. Nicolato**** and L. Casentini[†]

*Division of Neurosurgery, Padova, Italy
**Unit of Biostatics and Epidemiology, Fidia Lbs,
Abano Terme, Italy
***Division of Neurosurgery, Treviso, Italy
****Department of Neurosurgery, Verona, Italy
[†]Division of Neurosurgery, Vicenza, Italy

INTRODUCTION

Primary malignat brain tumors constitute only about 2% of all cancer in humans. Glioma occur with an incidence of 4.7 per 100.000 population (Walkeret et al, 1985). However they are an important cause of cancer morbidity and mortality. In addition, treatment of brain tumor has not significantly improved survival in recent years. Many patients who do survive more than 5 years are left with permanent disabilities.

Despite the importance of the morbidity and mortality associated with brain tu - mors, relatively little is known about risk factors or possible, causative agents associated with development of these tumors, although both genetic and environmental factors have been implicated.

This paper will review the literature on epidemiological investigation of brain glioma to summarize what is known about their etiology, associated risk factors and possible mechanism of brain tumor induction.

ETIOLOGICAL HYPOTHESES

Theories as to the origin of neoplasm of the central nervous system may be divided into two major categories: 1) the embryogenic cell-rest hypothesis, and 2) the hypothesis considering neoplastic transformation of normal adult cells or of congenital susceptible "cell-rest" under certain environmental influences. Such environmental factors may be diverse, viral or parasitic infection, chemical intoxication, trauma and other agents attributable to metabolic disturbance and mutation of nervous cells.

REVIEW OF EPIDEMIOLOGAL LITERATURE

Available epidemiological studies and their contribution as to the possible correlation (positive, negative or controversial) with development of brain tumors by several agents are summarized in table 1 and 2 that collect congenital and environmental factors.

PRESENTATION OF A NEW EPIDEMIOLOGICAL STUDY AND BASIC CRITERIA FOR PREPARATION OF THE WORKING PROTOCOL

Additional studies on the epidemiology of cerebral glioma are prompted by at least two reasons, that is the search of their etiology and of environmental risk
factors.
In this study epidemiological investigation is limited to cerebral glioma in a -
dults with exclusion of other typer of brain tumors.
Another important and basic aspects of the study is the definition of a limited
numbers of factors investigated, selected from the many possible ones, in order
to extensively explore the influence of these agents, without expanding beyond
certain limits the bulk of collected informations.
In fact, if protocol is expanded and filled with too many factors studied, there
is the risk of carrying a superficial investigation or of burdening the protocol
to a maximum of practical unfeasibility which would humper the final results.
The criteria of choce among the various possible etiological factors were a compromise between personal convinction and controversial results reported in the
literature. When convincing evidence of positive or negative correlation with the
development of glioma was reported for a certain factor, then the factor was excluded from our protocol.
In our questionary the following risk factors are investigated, each of which is
assigned a different lenght of space with various number of explorative questions
The factors are enlisted according to their relevance:
1) Familial aggregation
2) Head trauma
3) Radiations
4) Viral infections
5) ABO blood group
6) Chronic diseases
7) Drugs
8) Environmental,social and occupational factors

CONCLUSION

Thus far, few epidemiological approaches to the problem have been made and few
clues have been provided as to the origin of brain glioma. For these reasons the
authors decided to design and conduct a new epidemiological study of brain glioma, which is a multifactorial case-control study restricted to primary glioma in
adults. This study starts as a cooperative program of the Veneto Region in con-
junction with its four neurosurgical centers of Padova, Treviso, Verona and Vicenza.

TABLE 1   CONGENITAL FACTORS

TYPE	CONCLUSIVE RESULTS	AUTHORS
Race	– higher frequency of glioma in American Caucasians than in American Negroes (p$<$0.005)	Heshmat et al. 1976, Fan et al 1977
	– brain tumors more frequent in whites than non-whites (ratio = 1.5)	Gold 1980
Sex	– higher incidence of gliomas in males than in females M/F ratio = 1.36 : 1 M/F ratio = 7.21 : 6.76 M/F ratio = 6.2 : 4.9	Choi et al 1970 Barker et al. 1976 Kurland et al 1982
Familial Aggregation	– several occasional cases reported without statistical support	Kjellin et al 1960, Metzel 1964, Armstrong et al.1969, Kaufman et al. 1972, Isamat et al 1974, Schoenberg et al 1975, Schianchi et al 1980, Todd et al, 1981, Chadduck et al 1982, Wold et al 1982, Challa et al 1983 Farwell et al 1984, Janisch et al 1984, Maroun et al 1984, Saleman et al 1984, Sato et al 1984, Lesnick et al 1985.
Chromosome Studies	– no chromosomal abnormalities	Chadduck et al 1982
ABO blood group	– higher incidence of type A blood in glioma cases than in controls	Gaisford et al 1958, Yates et al 1960, Selverston et al 1961.
	– no significant differences	Buckwalter et al 1959, Garcia et al 1963, Choi et al 1970

TABLE 2   ENVIRONMENTAL FACTORS

TYPE	CONCLUSIVE RESULTS	AUTHORS
Radiations	– positive correlation after radiotherapy for tinea capitis	– Albert et al 1968, Modan et al 1974, Shore et al 1976
	– 2 personal cases of glioblastoma after irradiation for pituitary adenoma and 14 cases collected from the literature.	– Piatt et al 1983
	– 1 case of postirradiation cerebellar glioma	– Raffel et al 1985
Working Environment	Positive correlation in – farmers – veterinarians – nuclear workers – chemical workers	– Choi et al 1970, Musicco et al 1982 – Blair et al 1982 – Hadjimichael et al 1983 – Tabershaw et al 1974, Byren et al 1976, Waxweiler et al 1976, Reeve et al 1981, Werner et al 1981
	– pharmaceutical workers – rubber workers	– Thomas et al 1979, Olin et al 1980 – McMichael et al 1974, Mancuso 1976, Monson et al 1978
	– petrolchemical workers	– Theriault et al 1979, Thomas et al 1979, Reeve et al 1982, Leffingwell et al 1983, Waxveiler et al 1983

(%)

(% TAB. 2)

ENVIRONMENTAL FACTORS

TYPE	CONCLUSIVE RESULTS	AUTHORS
Head trauma	Incidence of glioblastoma markedly increased in severe head injury (p=0.004)	– Hochberg et al 1984
	No correlation	– Choi et al 1970, Annegers et al 1979, Kurland et al 1982
Neurological diseases	Epilepsy	– Choi et al 1970, Gold 1980, Mochberg et al 1984
	Multiple sclerosis	– Vierrege et al 1984
	Neurofibromatosis	– Brady 1962, Rodriguez et al 1966
	Tuberous sclerosis	– Rudnick et al 1961, Kapp et al 1967, Cooper 1971
Infections diseases	Toxoplasmosis	– Shuman et al 1967
	Tubercolisis	– Ward et al 1973
Smoking and alcohol	no correlation	– Choi et al 1970, Musicco et al 1982

REFERENCES

Albert R.E., and Omran A.R. (1968). Arch. Environ. Health, 17, 899-918
Annegers J.F., Kurkand L.T., Grabow J.D., Groover R.V., and Lews E.R. Jr. (1979).
   Neurology, 29, 578
Armstrong R.M., and Hanson C.W. (1969). Neurology, 19, 1061-1063
Barker D.J.P., Weller R.O. and Garfield J.S. (1976). J. Neurol. Neuros. Psych.
   39, 290-296.
Blair A., and Hayes Jr. H.M. (1982). Intern. J. of Epidem., 11 , 391-397.
Brady W.J. (1962). J. Neuropathol.Exp. Neurol., 21, 555-565
Buckwalter J.A., Turner J.H., Gamber H.H., Ratemar L., Saper R.T., and Knowler
   L.A. (1959). A.A.A. Arch. Neurol. Psychiatr., 81, 480-488
Byren D., Engholm G., Englund A., and Westerholm P. (1976). Envir. Health Persp.
   17 , 167-170.
Chadduck W.N., and Netsky M.G. (1982). Neurosurg., 10, 445-449.
Challa V.R., Goodman H.O., Davis C.H. (1983). Neurosurg., 12, 18-22.
Choi N.M., Schuman L.M., and Gullen W.H. (1970). Am.J.Epidemiol., 91, 238-259
Choi N.M., Schuman L.M., and Gullen W.H. (1970). Am. J.Epidemiol., 91, 467-485
Cooper J.R. (1971). J. Neurosurg., 34 , 194-202.
Fan K.J., Kovi J., and Earle (1977). J. Neuropatho. Exp. Neurol., 36, 41-49
Farwell J.R., Dohrmann G.J., and Flannery J.T. (1984). J. Neurosurg.,61,657-664
Gaisford W., and Compbell A.C.P. (1958). 36th Annual Report, Part. I-II, 533-538
Garcia J.H., Okazaki H., Aronson S.M. (1963). J. Neurosurg., 20, 397-399.
Gold E.B. (1980). Rev. in Canc. Epidemiol. 245-292.
Hadjimichael O.C., Ostefeld A.M., D'Atri D.A., and Brubaker R.E. (1983). J. Occu-
   pat. Medic., 25
Heshmat M.Y., Kovi J., Simpson C., Kennedy J., and Fan K.J. (1976). Cancer, 38
   2135-2142.
Hochberg F., Toniolo P., and Cole P. (1984). Neurol., 34, 1511-1514.
Isamat F., Miranda A.M., Bartumeus F., and Prat J. (1974). J. Neurosurg., 41,
   573-575.
Janisch W., Haas J.F., Schreiber D., and Gerlach M. (1984). J. Neuro-Ocol.,2
   113-116.
Kapp J.P., Paulson G.W., and Odom G.L. (1967). J. Neurosurg., 26 , 191-202.
Kaufman H.H., Brisman R. (1972). J. Neurosurg., 37, 110-112.
Kjellin K., Müller R., and Aström K.E. (1960). J. Neuropath. Exp. Neurol., 19,
   528-537.
Kurland L.T., Molgaard C.A., and Schoenberg B.S. (1982). Neuroepidemiol. 1,
   102-114.
Leffingwell S.S., Waxweiler R., Alexander V., Ludwig H.R.,and Halperin W.(1983).
   Neuroepidemiol., 2, 179-195.
Lesnick J.E., Chayt K.J., Bruce D.A., Rorke L.B., Trojanowski J., Savino P.J.,
   Schatz N.J. (1985). J. Neurosurg., 62, 930-932.
Mancuso T.F. (1976). Envir. Health Perspect., 17 , 21-30.
Maroun F.B., Jacob J.C., Heneghan W.D., Mangan M.A., Russel N.A., Ali S.K., Mur-
   rat G.P., and Clarke A. (1984). Surg. Neurol., 22 , 76-78.
McMichael A.J., Spirtas R., and Kupper L.L. (1974). J. Occup. Med., 16 , 458-464.
Metzel E. (1964). Acta Genet.Med. Gemellol., 13 , 124-131.
Modan B., Mart H., Baidatz D., Steinitz R., and Levin S.G. (1974). The Lancet,23,
   277-279.

Monson R.R., and Fine L.J. (1978). J.N.C.I., 61, 1047-1053.

Musicco M., Filippini G., Bordo B.M., Melotto A., Morello G., and Berrino F. (1982). Amer.J. of Epidemiol., 16, 782-790.

Olin G.R., and Ahlbom A. (1980). Environ. Res., 22, 154-161.

Piatt J.M., Blue J.M., Schold S.C., and Burger P.C. (1983). Neurosurg.,13,85-89.

Raffel C., Edwards M.S.B., Davis R.L., and Ablin A.R. (1985). J. Neurosurg., 62 300-303.

Reeve G.R., Lloyd J.W., and Alexander V. (1981). Ann. NY Acad.Sci., 381, 62-72.

Reeve G.R., Thomas T.L., Kelly V.F., Waxweiler R.J., and Itawa S. (1982). Ann. NY Acad. Sci., 381 , 54-61.

Rodriguez H.A., Berthrong M. (1966). Arch. Neurol., 14, 467-475.

Rudnick P.A., Hoshino N., and Kitaoka T. (1961), JAMA, 178 , 73-75.

Saleman M., and Solomon L. (1984). Neurosurg., 14, 557-561.

Sato T., Shimoda A., Takahashi T., Kurokawa H., Ando M., Goto S., and Takamura H. (1984). Child's Brain, 11, 342-348.

Schianchi P., and Kraus-Rupper R. (1980). Acta Neuropathol.,52, 153-155.

Schoenberg B.S., Glista G.G., and Reagan T.J. (1975). Surg. Neurol., 3, 139-145.

Schuman L.M., Choi N.W., and Gullen W.N. (1967). Am. J. Pub. Hlth., 57, 848-856.

Selverston B., and Cooper D.R. (1961). J. Neurosurg., 18 , 602-604.

Shore R.E., Albert R.E., and Pasternack B.S. (1976). Arch. Environ. Health, 31 21-28.

Tabershaw I.R., and Gaffey W.R. (1974). J. Occupat. Med., 16, 509-518.

Theriault G., and Goulet L. (1979). J. Occup. Med., 21, 367-370.

Thomas T.L., and Decoufle P. (1979). J. Occup. Med., 9 , 619-623.

Todd D.W., Christoferson L.A., Leech R.W., and Rudolf L. (1981). Ann. Neurol., 10, 390-392.

Vieregge P., Nahser H.C., Reinhardt V., Gerhard L., and Nau E. (1984). Cl. Neuropath., 3, 10-21.

Wald S.L., Liwnicz B.H., Truman T.A., and Khodadad G. (1982). Neurosurg.,11, 12-15.

Walker A.E., Robins M., and Weinfeld F.D. (1985). Neurol., 35, 219-226.

Ward D.W., Mattison M.L., and Finn R. (1983). Brit. Med. J.,1 , 83-84.

Waxweiler R.J., Stringer W., Wagoner J.K., Jones J., Falk H., and Carter C. (1976). Ann. NY Acad. Sci., 271, 40-48.

Waxweiler J., Victor A., Leffingwell S.S., Haring M., and Lloyd W. (1983). JNCI, 70, 75-81.

Werner J.B., and Carter J.T. (1981). Br.J.Ind.Med., 38, 247-253.

Yates P.O., and Pearce K.M. (1960). Lacet, 1, 194-195.

Therapy for Central Nervous System Malignant Tumors

P. Paoletti, R. Knerich, D. Adinolfi, G. Butti
and S. Pezzotta

Department of Surgery, Neurosurgical Section, Centre
"E. Grossi-Paoletti" for Study and Treatment of Nervous System
Tumors, University of Pavia, Italy

ABSTRACT

Although in recent years a great attempt has been made in brain tumor therapy
it appears to be conditioned by a large number of problems such as cell
kinetics, tumor growth modalities, presence of blood-brain barrier, drug
delivery, a.s.o.. Surgery play only an important role but a complete removal
of the tumor mass may be considered only palliative from a theoretic point of
view. Therefore, surgical procedure can be palliative for neurologic symptoms,
give an accurate diagnosis, and appropriate time to administer adjuvant
therapies. These latter therapeutic approaches, namely radiotherapy and chemotherapy, can be of relevance in prolonging survival of operated patients.
Radiotherapy must be performed at the maximum tolerable dose (60 Gy whole
brain) but, if optimal results have been obtained, a lot of drawbacks,
primarily the increase of necrosis in normal brain, were observed. Nor "two
volume radiation "(45 Gy whole brain, 10-15 Gy on the tumoral bed), nor
applications of radiosensitizers, nor daily dose superfractionation or local
hypertermia demonstrate any better survival than conventional treatment. The
most effective chemotherapeutic agent is certainly BCNU. Clinical, biochemical
and biopathological studies support this regimen. Some other drugs, such as
CCNU, ACNU, PCNU, streptozotocin, and procarbazine are of same value in
treating brain malignancies but toxicity appears the major dose limiting
problem. The future of chemotherapy appears to be related to disposal of new
drugs, to different times or routes of administration, and to combination of
drugs. Finally, immunotherapy raises the same and other problems. In fact,
immunoreaction was demostrated inside the brain and malignancies but, unfortunately, current immunotherapy agents are unable to produce significant improvements in survival of patients with brain tumors.

KEYWORDS

Malignant brain tumors, surgery, radiotherapy, chemotherapy, immunotherapy.

INTRODUCTION

The problems related to malignant brain tumor therapy are: tumor factors, host-to-tumor factors, host factors and independent factors.
Cell kinetic and tumor cell distribution are the principal tumor factors; blood brain barrier (BBB), the host-to-tumor factor; age, sex, performance status and tumor location, the host factors; support therapy and criteria for definition of response to treatment and recurrence, the independent factors.
Surgery, radiotherapy, chemotherapy and immunotherapy are therapeutic modalities for a combined treatment of malignant gliomas. Such a multidisciplinary approach has both beneficial aspects and limits. All of them must be kept in mind in order to avoid effects that any single treatment may have on other.

SURGERY

Surgery plays an important role in brain tumor therapy. The goals of brain tumor surgery are summarized in table 1.

TO MAKE DIAGNOSIS

TO PERFORM CYTOREDUCTIVE THERAPY

TO TREAT SYMPTOMS

TO PROVIDE TIME TO ADMINISTER
OTHER THERAPIES

TO ALTER TUMOR CELL KINETICS

TABLE 1.   Goals of malignant brain tumor
surgery.

Surgery provides tissue for histological examination that is the most effective means for accurate diagnosis and tumor treatment. Secondly, surgical removal of the tumor mass may be the only method for reducing pressure on surrounding tissue consequently removing unwanted symptoms. Surgery is the only therapy which removes tumor cells. Surgical resection does not always offer a cure for tumors, but at least it can prolong a patient's life and give more time for adjuvant therapies. Resection of a tumor mass causes quiescent cells to enter an active growth phase, thus making them more susceptible targets of radiation and chemotherapy.
Proliferating cells, resting cells, sterile and dead cells are the four components that make up a tumor mass. The goal of brain tumor surgery is for the complete removal of these cells, but the invasion of proliferating cells into the healthy part of the brain adjacent to the tumor (BAT) prevents this possibility of becoming a reality (Ransohoff 1979, Garfield 1980, Paoletti et al. 1981, Paoletti 1984, Paoletti and Butti 1984).
Survival of patients with malignant brain tumors is affected by different clinical factors. Some variables significantly decrease the death rate after surgery. They are: patient age (less than 45 years), histopathologic cathegory (anaplastic astrocytoma), performance status (70 or more), ABO blood type (B and 0), pre-treatment wbc count (more than 5,500/mm^3), pre-treatment platelet count (200,000/mm^3 or more), duration of symptoms (more than 6 months) and

consciousness level (Green et al 1983).
However, if treatment is limited to only surgery modest results are obtained.
Total removal plus lobectomy has been found to markedly increase survival time
with respect to simple surgical or stereotactic biopsy (Paoletti and Butti
1984). The median survival time is in fact only 17 weeks in the latter case
(Walker et al 1978) even if the optimal tumor burden reduction possibility by
surgery is 2 log cell kill, that is the decrease of the tumor weight from 100
g. to 1 g. and of the number of cells from 10^{11} to 10^9.
The quality of life may be improved by treating the surrounding brain edema.
Hyperventilation, ventricular drainage, diuretics, corticosteroids and barbitu-
rates may be extremely useful (Knerich et al. 1980, 1985).

RADIOTHERAPY

The first report from the Brain Tumor Study Group (BTSG) of the U.S. National
Cancer Institute showed that radiotherapy, when applied at about 60 Gy whole
brain on patients operated for malignant brain tumors increased median survival time to 37.5 weeks from the 17 obtained from surgery alone (Walker et al.
1978, Paoletti 1984);
Later studies of the BTSG demonstrated that doses of less than 50 Gy have
little effect as does limited irradiation of the tumor mass, even when given
in high doses (Walker et al. 1978, Green et al. 1983).
Beneficial results of radiation therapy at high doses are: a net decrease in
cell proliferation with a reduction in the number of mitosis, macrophagic stimulation and vascular alterations.
Despite this, there are a number of drawbacks, primarily the increase of necrosis in normal brain tissue. To avoid these toxic side effects recent proposals
concerning radiotherapy have been to reduce the dose to 45 Gy whole brain
associated with a 10-15 Gy to the tumor only. In this way, normal brain tissue
would receive a tolerable dose while the amount focused on the tumor mass
would be therapeutically useful (Knerich et al. 1985).
One of the main obstacles of radiotherapy for malignant brain tumors is the
presence of hypoxic cells. To get around this problems various alternatives
have been suggested, such as varying dose and fractionation other than 1.8-2
Gy/day, 1 fraction/day, 5 days a week for 6 to 7 weeks, and using radiosensitizers and heat.
Another solution is superfractionated daily doses. This tecnique is based on
the concept that normal cells tend to shield themselves better and faster than
tumor cells from sub-lethal demage caused by ionized radiation (Shapiro 1982,
Paoletti and Knerich 1983).
Radiosensitizers have been suggested in order to obtain an adequate oxygenation
of tumor cells during radiotherapy (Sheline et al. 1979). Hyperbaric oxygen (3
atm.) has proven effective and, recently, so have nitromidazole derivatives,
particularly misonidazole. Analogous results can be obtained with a combination
of radiotherapy and local hypertermia, bringing the temperature of the brain
tumor to 43°C while maintaining normal brain tissue at 40°C or less (Salcman
and Samaras 1981).
The optimal tumor burden reduction by radiotherapy added to surgery is another
2 log cell kill, which would decrease the tumor weight to 1/10000 and the
number of tumor cells from 10^7 to 10^5.

CHEMOTHERAPY

The most promising approach to malignant gliomas in the last decade was chemotherapy. Chemotherapy must take into account drug-related problems such as chemical and pharmacological characteristics, oncolytic mode of action, pharma-cokinetics, potential cell kill, route and the timing of administration, pres-ence of resistant cells, DNA-repair mechanisms and toxicity. Cell kinetics of gliomas and the presence of the BBB are also of primary importance.

Using several different methods, Hoshino et al. (1975, 1977) have calculated the kinetic parameters of experimental and human brain tumors. In comparison to the majority of other solid tumors, malignant gliomas have a lower growth fraction (30-40%) and a higher cell loss (80-90%). The duration of S phase is 4.4-10.5 hours (and these values are common to anaplastic astrocytoma and glioblastoma) and a doubling time of 45-55 days if cell loss factor is consi-dered.

These kinetic data have important implications for the selection of drugs effective in brain tumors. In fact, because of the small number of viable cycling cells, if a cell-cycle-specific (CCS) agent is used, only 30-40% of tumor cell population will be affected by this drug and, with few exceptions, only those cells which are in one phase (usually the S phase) of the cell cycle die. This oncolytic effect would permit only 10% reduction of tumor diameter. Furthermore, tumor size could be poorly affected because of retarded dead cell removal and prompt tumor repopulation due to recruitment of cells from a non-proliferating pool. Therefore, cell-cycle-non-specific (CCNS) drugs seem to be the most effective agents in treating these tumors.

Drug delivery, pharmacologic and pharmacokinetic problems are also of great importance in brain tumor chemotherapy. Normal brain capillaries exclude non ionized hydrophilic molecules with a molecular weight (M.W.) greater than 180 whereas, within particular physical limits of lipophilicity and molecular size (lipid/aqueous ratio smaller than 30 and M.W. lower than 480), the BBB transport of lipophilic drug is quite rapid and, for many substances, limited only by blood flow (Levin 1979).

Proceeding from the tumor core to BAT the capillaries of malignant brain tumors progressively contain a smaller number of imperfect interendothelial junctions, perforations, destructions and other abnormalities, the result of which is the BBB disruption. The major part of the tumor (core and, in some location, also growing edge) has a BBB partially or completely disrupted whereas BAT (which contains infiltrating cells) has a limited capillary permea-bility. This anatomical configuration implies that drugs which cross the normal BBB (such as lipid soluble, poorly ionized and with low M.W.) reach a similar concentration in the tumor and in the BAT.

From these considerations it is obvious that a drug like BCNU (i.e. CCNS, which cross the BBB) is of greater value in treating malignant brain tumors than CCS or hydrophilic drug (i.e. Bleomycin, 5-Fluorouracil, Methotrexate, etc.) (Levin and Wilson 1976, Levin 1979).

Some nitrosourea compounds (BCNU, CCNU, ACNU, PCNU), streptozotocin and procar-bazine are, at present, the most effective drugs in treating brain malignancies both in adult patients and in children.

The response rate ranges between 40 and 50% of treated patients (Walker et al. 1978, 1980, Paoletti et al. 1979).

Several new drugs (Cis-platinum, VM-26, VP-16, Triazinate, Chlorozotocin, Dianhydrogalactitol, etc.) are presently under evaluation (Shapiro and Byrne 1983).

Table 2 shows perspective, controlled and randomized clinical trials of adju-vant monochemotherapy after surgery. These studies were made from 1971 to

AUTHOR	TREATMENT	No. PTS	MEDIAN SURVIVAL (wks)
Edland et al. (1971)	RT RT+5-FU	30	49 50
Armentrout et al. (1974)	RT RT+BCNU	27	30 43
Weir et al. (1976)	RT CCNU RT+CCNU	41	27 37 36
Reagan et al. (1976)	RT CCNU RT+CCNU	63	50 28 52
EORTC (1978)	RT+CCNU (early) RT+CCNU (late)	81	43 62
Paoletti et al. (1979)	RT+BCNU RT+CCNU	126	54 50
Solero et al. (1979)	RT RT+BCNU RT+CCNU	102	46 56 74

RT: radiotherapy
5-FU: 5-fluorouracil
BCNU: 1,3 bis (2-chloroethyl)-1-nitrosourea
CCNU: 1-(2-chloroethyl)-3-cyclohexyl-1-nitrosourea

TABLE 2. Prospective, controlled and randomized clinical
trials of adjuvant monochemotherapy after surgery.

1979. Table 3 shows the results of the BTSG obtained from 1976 to 1984.
The results obtained clearly demonstrate that surgery plus radiotherapy and
BCNU is the best treatment available. Procarbazine and streptozotocin give
similar results. Mithramycin and methylprednisolone have no effects and fractionated radiotherapy or the addition of misonidazole as a radiosensitizer are
not able to improve the results obtained with conventional radiotherapy.
New approaches to brain tumor chemotherapy now under investigation are: route
of administration (intraarterial for BCNU and Cis-platinum); high doses of
BCNU with bone marrow rescue; drugs after osmotic BBB disruption; time of
administration (in relation to surgery); different drugs in different times.
Some Authors (Tel et al. 1980), using a brain tumor experimental model, have
shown that survival time increased when BCNU was given 1 hour before or 1 to
12 hours after surgery.
Based on these results, we designed in 1982 a pilot study which called for
administration of BCNU 6 to 8 hours after surgery at a dose of 220 mg/m^2 i.v.
Radiotherapy was started within three weeks after surgery. The scheduled dose
was 45 Gy whole brain with a boost of 15 Gy on the tumor bed delivered over a
period of 6 to 7 weeks. Chemotherapy courses were repeated every 8 weeks
(Butti et al. 1984).
From April 1982 to June 1983, 24 non-selected patients were entered into the

| | | | MEDIAN SURVIVAL |
AUTHOR	TREATMENT	No.PTS	(wks)
WALKER et al.	Controls	96	26
(1976)	Mithramycin		21
WALKER et al.	Controls		17
(1978)	BCNU	303	25
	RT		37.5
	RT+BCNU		40.5
WALKER et al.	RT+BCNU		50.3
(1980)	MeCCNU	349	31
	RT		36
	RT+MeCCNU		34.6
GREEN et al.	RT+BCNU		50
(1983)	RT+Methylprednisolone	609	40
	RT+PCZ		47
	RT+BCNU+Methylprednisolone		41
GREEN et al.	RT+BCNU		45
(1984)	RT+STZ	557	45
	Fractionated RT+BCNU		45
	RT+misonidazole+BCNU		45

MeCCNU = methyl-CCNU
PCZ   = procarbazine
STZ   = streptozotocin

TABLE 3. Prospective, controlled and randomized clinical studies of adjuvant
monochemotherapy after surgery. Results from the Brain Tumor Study
Group (NCI).

study. 21 were evaluable: 2 patients were excluded because lost to follow-up
and one patient's histopathological review showed a metastasis.
There were 13 males and 8 females and the average age was 53 with a range from
17 to 70 years. 71.5% of the patients have glioblastoma. The most involved
area was the temporal lobe.
A gross total removal was done in 6 cases and a subtotal in 15. The percentage
of survivors at different interval is detailed in table 4. Six months from
beginning of treatment all patients were alive. 38% have survived for two
years. The median survival time is 16.6 months. Toxic effects were nausea,
vomiting, burning at the injection site, leukopenia and thrombocytopenia,
which did not differ from our previous experience. In one patient the
treatment was discontinued after the sixth cycle because of severe hematologic
toxicity. There have been no signs of pulmonary fibrosis.
Promising results in treating tumors with drugs have been obtained by using a
combination of agents as opposed to one only (Table 5). The success of

INTERVAL FROM SURGERY (mos)	SURVIVAL
6	100%
12	62%
18	48%
24	38%
30	14%

TABLE 4: Final evaluation of survival of BCNU chemotherapy started immediately after surgery.

combined chemotherapy in treating other solid tumors would appear to constitute a valid reason for its application in malignant brain tumor therapy.
We designed a clinical pilot study of combined chemotherapy in 1978. From November 1978 to June 1981 20 patient with recurrent malignant glioma aged over 15 years underwent combined chemotherapy: CCNU (120 mg/m^2 D1), VM-26 (100 mg/m^2 D2-4), and 5-FU (450 mg/m^2 D10-14).
Each cycle was repeated every 6-8 weeks. 14/20 patients were evaluable: 8 patients were responders to therapy, 3 non-responders and 3 were classified as partial responder. Median survival was 51.3 weeks in reponders (median duration of response: 40 weeks) and 19.6 weeks in non-responders (Knerich et al. 1981). Nausea, vomiting and hair loss were the most frequent non-hematologic drug-related toxic effects. One patient developed a severe idiosyncratic reaction to VM-26 after the 9th cycle of therapy and in another patient a serious liver impairment was determined after the 4th course of treatment; the hematologic toxicity was low.
Considering the total amount of drugs delivered, the WBC and PLT count nadir were generally acceptable (Robustelli della Cuna et al, 1982).
On the basis of this study, a phase III protocol was activated in March 1984 in which patients with primitive malignant glioma are randomized, after surgery, to Rt + CCNU vs. Rt + CCNU + VM-26 vs. Rt + CCNU + VM-26 + 5-FU.
Eligibility criteria are as follows: patients with primary malignant gliomas; age not under 15 yrs.; supratentorial location of the tumor; Karnofsky score not less than 30; surgical procedure other than biopsy; no major medical, neurological, or psichiatric illness (other than glioma); no previous surgical, radiological, or chemotherapeutic treatment of primary; refusal of treatment (patient or his family).
Assigned treatment starts within 3 weeks from surgery. Scheduled doses of RT are 45 Gy whole brain and 10-15 Gy on the tumoral bed, delivered over 6-7 weeks Chemotherapy is administered at 8 week intervals and standard dose of each drug is reduced or the treatment discontinued if toxicity develops.
Since the aim of this study are to determine if combined versus single agent chemotherapy could be of greater value in prolonging survival of patients bearing malignant gliomas, almost 200 evaluable patients will be considered over 3 to 4 years. Time consumed for follow-up evaluation will be approximately one year.
On June 1, 1985, 48 patients entered into the study, 46 of which were eligible. The population is characterized as follows: male/female ratio equal to 1; mean age 59 yrs. with a range of 21 to 75; histologic diagnosis of glioblastoma in 50% of cases, anaplastic astrocytoma in 46%; in two patients a gliosarcoma was found. Location of these tumors is primarily on right side (54%) and frontal and temporal lobe are the most involved areas.
Surgery was performed in all patients. Gross total or subtotal resection of the tumor mass was obtained in approximately 30% of the patients. In many

AUTHOR	TREATMENT	No.OF CASES	R (%)	MEDIAN DURATION (wks)	
				FREE INTERVAL	SURVIVAL
FEWER et al. (1972)	BCNU+VCR	20	25	23	--
HILDEBRAND et al. (1973)	CCNU+VCR+MTX	16	25	37	53
TAYLOR et al. (1975)	DTIC+CCNU+MeCCNU	16	19	12	32
GUTIN et al. (1975)	PCZ+VCR+CCNU	30	--	39	--
POUILLART et al. (1976)	ADM+VM26+CCNU	43	72	--	26
LEVIN et al. (1976)	BCNU+PCZ	45	47	34	--
CANDRY et al. (1978)	VCR+VM26+CCNU	38	47	13	--
HEISS et al. (1978)	Methylidrazine+ CTX+5-FU+MTX+ Methylprednisolone	27	--	23	38
LEVIN et al. (1978)	BCNU+5-FU	29	31	34	25
LEVIN et al. (1979)	BCNU+HU	27	--	42	--
AVELLANOSA et al. (1979)	MeCCNU+VCR+PCZ	28	32	25	--
SEILER et al. (1980)	Prednisone+CCNU	27	55	--	58

R: Response to treatment.
DTIC = Dacarbazine; VCR = Vincristine; MTX = Methotrexate; ADM = Adriamycin;
VM-26 = Teniposide; CTX = Cyclophosphamide; HU = Hydroxyurea

TABLE 5. Polychemotherapy in the treatment of malignant brain tumors.

cases this surgical accomplishment was associated to lobectomy. The mean number of given courses of chemotherapy was 4 with a dose reduction in only advanced cycles.

IMMUNOTHERAPY

Numerous research protocols have been devised for the purpose of showing immuno-therapy effectiveness, both specific and aspecific. In active specific immuno therapy the substances utilized, from an antigenic stand point, are correlated to the tumor. These substances should stimulate a specific and selective immune response in the host. To this end tumor cells (also in a homogeneized form) are one of the substances employed. They are first inactivated with radiation or antiblastic treatment. Another product used is viral or bacterial cross-reacting antigens and, a third substance employed is tumor antigens (Apuzzo and Mitchell 1981).
In active aspecific immunotherapy, where the object is to increase the host's immunoreactivity in an aspecific way, the substances employed have no antigenic affinity with the tumor. The most commonly used substances are Corynebacterium Parvum and the bacillus Calmett-Guèrin (BCG). We used this last in a randomized study combined with radiotherapy and chemotherapy with nitrosourea derivatives (BCNU, CCNU), but with unsatisfactory results (Table 6) (Butti et al. 1983).

TREATMENT	No.PTS	MEDIAN SURVIVAL (wks)	P
Surgery & RT +BCNU	16	47	*
Surgery & RT +BCNU + BCG	15	45	NS
RT + CCNU	11	35	*
RT + CCNU + BCG	11	34	NS

NS = Not significant. (Wilcoxon test)

TABLE 6. BCG aspecific active immunotherapy of malignant brain tumors.

Recently, interferons have been used in the treatment of malignant brain tu-mors. It has been administered systemically or into the lesion in small groups of patients with transient beneficial responses having been reported by some authors (Nagai et al. 1983, Boethius et al. 1983). Mahaley et al. (1983) poin-ted out that administration of interferon could represent an alternative to the use of BCNU as an adjunct in the management of anaplastic gliomas.

CONCLUSIONS

Despite some improvement in the lenght and quality of survival, the majority of patients with malignant brain tumors die within two years from treatment. Death is usually cerebral, characterized by a progression of neurological sym-ptoms all traceable to the impossibility of completely eradicating the primi-tive lesion. When a patient develops a brain tumor his skull, which normally contains 1200 ml., becomes restricted. In such a restricted space 100 g of tumor, equivalent to 100 billion cells, are lethal.

Patients presenting evident symptoms, who are examined by a neurosurgeon for
the first time, usually have a tumor of about 60-80 g. Assuming that the brain
tumor weighs 100 g (100 billion cells), a gross total surgical resection can
remove a maximum of 99% of the tumor (2 log cell kill) leaving 1 g or 1
billion cells. Radiation therapy may further reduce the tumor mass to about 2
log, bringing it to 0.01 g (10 million cells).
Chemotherapy is asked to decrease the tumor cell population to 0.0001 g
(10,000 cells), which is a size that the host's immunological system can
destroy. However, surgery is usually unable to destroy more than 2 log, while
chemotherapy can generally destroy 1-2 log (Table 7) (Sano 1983).

	REDUCTION POSSIBILITY	WEIGHT (g)	No.OF CELLS
TUMOR (diagnosis)	--	100	10^{11}
SURGERY	2 LOG	1	10^{9}
RADIOTHERAPY	2 LOG	0.01	10^{7}
CHEMOTHERAPY	2 LOG	0.0001	10^{5}
IMMUNOTHERAPY	?	?	?

TABLE 7. Optimal burden reduction possibilities by different therapeutic modalities.

It is therefore extremely improbable to cure a person with a malignant brain
tumor. This possibility is calculated to be about 1 out of 10.000 cases
(Walker 1978).
Cytoreduction of the tumor causes the tumor to increase its growth more quikly
than it can be destroyed.
With its limits already defined, it appears unlikely that surgery will be able
to improve further. Thus, future prospects in treating these tumors may lie in
the improvement of results already obtained with radiotherapy and adjuvant
chemotherapy through the definition of the timing of radiotherapy, of the
correct dose and fractionation, of the possibility in the use of radiosensitizers, and the use of new sources of radiation. On the other hand, discovery of
effective new drugs and of sequences which take into account tumor biological
characteristics, is another important field where research may improve brain
tumor therapy. Lastly, problems of a certain relevance are: definition of
prognostic factors, criteria for evaluating response and the role played by
support therapy.
Immunotherapy may still offers further possibilities. In any case, there are
may and complex problems that must still be solved and correctly defined
before their place in combined malignant brain tumor therapy can be predicted.

ACKNOWLEDGEMENTS

These researches were supported in part by Contr. No. 84.00713.44, Special
Project "Oncologia", National Research Council, Rome, Italy.

REFERENCES

Apuzzo M.L.J., Mitchell M.S. (1981). J. Neurosurg. 55, 1-18.

Armentrout S.A., Folt E., Vermund H., Otis T.P. (1974). Cancer Chemother. Rep. 58, 841-844.

Avellanosa A.M., West C.R., Tsukada Y., Higby D.J., Bakshi S., Reege P.A., Jemmings E. (1979). Cancer 44, 839-842.

Boethius J., Blomgren M., Collins V.P. (1983). Acta Neurochir. 68, 239-251.

Butti G., Knerich R., Adinolfi D., Locatelli D., Paoletti P. (1983). Il Policlinico - Sez. Chir. 90, 1277-1280.

Butti G., Knerich R., Tanghetti B., Adinolfi D., Gaetani P., Buoncristiani P., Paoletti P. (1984). Cancer Treat. Rep. 68, 1505-1506.

Candry M., Guérin J., Celériér D., Baunayan M., Candry R., Constant P., Caille J.C., Pouyanne H., Reboul G. (1978). Bordeaux Medical 11, 1081-1089

Edland R.W., Javid M., Ansfield F.J. (1971). Am. J. Roentgenol. Radium Ther. Nucl. Med. 111, 337-343.

EORTC Brain Tumor Group. (1978). Eur. J. Cancer 14, 851-857.

Fewer D., Wilson C.B., Boldrey E.R., Enot K.J., Powell M.R. (1972). J.A.M.A. 222, 549-554.

Garfield J. (1980). In: Thomas D.G.T., Graham M.T. (eds.) - "Brain tumors". Butterworths - London, 301-321.

Green S.B., Byar D.P., Walker M.D., Pistenma D.A., Alexander E. jr., Batzdorf U., Brooks W.H., Hunt W.E., Mealey J.jr., Odom G.L., Paoletti P., Ransohoff J., Robertson J.T., Selker R.G., Shapiro W.R., Smith K.R., Wilson C.B., Strike T.A. (1983). Cancer Treat. Rep. 67, 121-132.

Green S.B., Byar D.P., Strike T.A., Alexander E. jr., Brooks W.H., Burger P.C., Hunt W.E., Mealey J., Odom G.L., Paoletti P., Pistenma D.A., Ransohoff J., Robertson J.T., Selker R.G., Shapiro W.R., Smith K.R. (1984). ASCO Proceedings, Toronto, May 6-8.

Gutin P.H., Wilson C.B., Kumar A.R.V., Boldrey E.B., Levin V.A., Powell M., Enot K.J. (1985). Cancer 35, 1398-1404.

Heiss W.D. (1978). Acta Neurochir. 42, 109-114.

Hildebrand J., Brihaye J., Wagenknecht C., Michel J., Kenis V. (1973). Eur. J. Cancer 9, 627-634.

Hoshino T., Wilson C.B. (1975). J. Neurosurg. 49, 13-21.

Hoshino T. (1977). Natl. Cancer Inst. Monogr. 46, 29-35.

Knerich R., Butti G., Bonezzi C., Introzzi G., Karussos G., Fraschini M., Caione A. (1980). Pharmacol. Res. Comm. 12, 899-908.

Knerich R., Tanghetti B., Locatelli D., Soffietti R. (1981). Neurochirurgia (Suppl.), 413.

Knerich R., Adinolfi D., Butti G., Pezzotta S., Soffietti R., Sciolla R., Vasario E., Pavesi L., Robustelli della Cuna G., Paoletti P., Schiffer D. (1985). Arg. Oncol. 6, 1-34.

Levin V.A. (1979). In: Paoletti P., Walker M.D., Butti G., Knerich R. (eds.) "Multidisciplinary Aspects of brain tumor therapy". Elsevier-Amsterdam, 165-172.

Levin V.A., Wilson C.B. (1976). In: Fewer D.A., Wilson C.B., Levin V.A. (eds.) - "Brain tumor chemotherapy" - C.C. Thomas - Springfield, Ill., 42-74.

Levin V.A., Grafts D.C., Wilson C.B., Schultz M.J., Boldrey E.B., Enot K.J., Pischer T.C., Seager M., Elashoff R.B. (1976). Cancer Treat. Rep. 60, 243-249.

Levin V.A., Hoffman V.F., Pischer T.L., Seager M.L., Boldrey E.B., Wilson C.B. (1978). Cancer Treat. Rep. 62, 2071 -2079.

Levin V.A., Wilson C.B., DavisR., Wara W.M., Pischer T.L., Irwin L. (1979). J. Neurosurg. 51, 526-532.

Mahaley M.S. jr., Urso M.B., Whaley R.A., Williams T.E., Guaspari A. (1984). J. Neurosurg. 61, 1069-1071.

Nagaj M., Arai T., Kohno S., Kohase M. (1982). In: Kono R., Vilcek J. (eds.) "The clinical potential of Interferons", Univ. of Tokio Press.

Paoletti P. (1984). J. Neurosurg. Sci. 28, 51-60.

Paoletti P., Butti G., Casotto A., Giunta F., Knerich R., Marini G., Mazza C., Robustelli della Cuna G., Schiffer D., Soffietti R. (1979). In: Paoletti P., Walker M.D., Butti G., Knerich R. (eds.) "Multidisciplinary aspects of brain tumor therapy" Elsevier-Amsterdam - 275-282.

Paoletti P., Brambilla G., Knerich R. (1981). In Giornate in onore del Maestro" - Soc. Medicina Sperimentale, Modena, 169-180.

Paoletti P., Knerich R. (1983). Med. Paz. 6, 24-33.

Paoletti P., Butti G. (1984). Min. Med. 75, 1305-1311.

Pouillart P., Mathé G., Thy T.H., Lheritier J., Poisson M., Huguenin P., Gautier H., Morin P., Parrot R. (1976). Cancer 38, 1909-1916.

Ransohoff J. (1979). In: Evans A.E. (ed.) "Modern Concepts in brain tumor therapy: laboratory and clinical investigations"-Castle House Publ. Ltd. - Beccles and London, 114-119.

Reagan T.J., Bisel H.F., Child D.S., Layton D.D., Rhoton A.L.jr., Taylor W.F. (1976). J. Neurosurg. 44, 186-190.

Robustelli della Cuna G., Paoletti P., Bernardo G., Knerich R., Butti G. Cuzzoni Q. (1982). Neurosurgery 11, 408-411.

Salcamn M., Samaras G.M. (1981). Neurosurgery 9, 327-335.

Sano K. (1983). Clinical Neurosurg. 30, 93-124.

Seiler R.W., Zimmerman A., Markwalder H. (1980). Surg.Neurol. 13, 65-70.

Shapiro W.R. (1982). Ann. Neurol. 12, 231-237.

Shapiro W.R., Byrne T.N. (1983). In: Walker M.D. (ed.) "Oncology of the nervous system" - Nijhoff M. - Boston - 65-100.

Sheline G., Wasserman T., Wara W., Phillips T. (1979). In: Paoletti P., Walker M.D., Butti G., Knerich R. (eds.) "Multidisciplinary Aspects of brain tumor therapy" - Elsevier-Amsterdam, 197-208.

Solero C.L., Monfardini S., Brambilla G., Vaghi A., Valagussa P., Bonadonna G., Morello G. (1979). Cancer Clin. Trials 2, 43-50.

Taylor S.G., Nelson L., Basker D., Rosenbaum L., Sponzo W.R., Cunnigham T.J., Olson K.B., Horton J. (1975). Cancer 36, 1269-1274.

Tel E., Hoshino T., Barker M.S. (1980). J. Neurosurg. 52, 529-532.

Walker M.D. (1978). In: Clin. Neurosurgery" 25 - Williams and Wilkins - Baltimore - 388-396.

Walker M.D., Alexander E. jr., Hunt W.E., Leventhal C.M., Mahaley M.S. jr., Mealey S. jr., Norrell H.A., Owens G., Ransohoff J., Wilson C.B., Gehan E.A. (1976) J. Neurosurg. 44, 655-667.

Walker M.D., Alexander E. jr., Hunt W., McCarthy C.S., Mahaley M.S.jr., Mealey J. jr., Norrel H.A., Owens G., Ransohoff J., Wilson C.B., Gehan E.A., Strike T.A. (1978). J.Neurosurg. 49, 333-343.

Walker M.D., Green S.B., Byar D.P., Alexander E. jr., Batzdorf V., Brooks W.H., Hunt W.E., McCarthy C.S., Mahaley M.S. jr., Mealy J.jr., Owens G., Ransohoff J., Robertson J.T., Shapiro W.R., Smith K.R. jr., Wilson C.B., Strike T.A. (1980). New Engl.J.Med. 303, 1323-1329.

Weir B., Band P., Urtasun R., Blain G., McLean D., Wilson F., Mielke B., Grace M. (1976). J. Neurosurg. 45, 129-134.

Closing Remarks

Our first neuro-oncological symposium, the 'Verona 1', is coming to an end. It sounds difficult indeed, to draw the conclusions of such an interesting meeting.

Brain tumors are not frequent, but their overall incidence is higher than commonly expected. In Italy, the National Oncological Register has shown in 1983-1984 an average of approximately 6000 new cases per year: 400 only in the Veneto Region.

Human and social costs of these diseases remain untolerably high. Fortunately, many of these are benign tumors, that can be safely treated and in most cases totally cured with presently available surgical and radiotherapic tools.

However, cerebral gliomas constitute more than 50% of all intracranial tumors. Quoting dr. Paul Bucy (Surg. Neurol. 1982)".. For over 100 years neurosurgeons have struggled with these neoplasms. To date the situation has improved. Surgical mortality and postoperative morbidity have been reduced, but the ultimate results remain the same as they were 100 years ago: all of the patients still die of their tumors. We have not learned how to cure them. This is discouraging and inexcusable. These are not 'malignant' tumors. They start in a localized area, and grow in a localized part of the brain. They do not metastasize. They do not develop in several areas, with rare exceptions. If they could be completely removed, those patients afflicted with them would be cured...".

It is our opinion that such an important task can be tackled only with the combined effort of basic researchers on one side, surgeons and clinicians on the other. This symposium has been designed to endorse this effort, creating a further opportunity for neuro-oncologists on both sides to meet and to confront ideas and experiences: we deem that the goal has been achieved.

Listening to acknowledged scientists and surgeons from leading international oncological centers, we had the feeling that even for these patients, quoting again dr. Bucy, "... there appears to be a light at the end of the tunnel".

With this deep belief we turn off the lights of this 'Verona 1', hoping to have you all here again in a near future for a continuing 'Verona 2'.

Massimo A. Gerosa
Mark L. Rosenblum
Giuseppe Tridente

Index

239